this book shine.
shopping and meal
free for patients embarking on the low-FODMAP diet."

— **Andrea Hardy, R.D., owner of Ignite Nutrition**

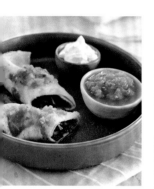
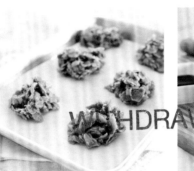
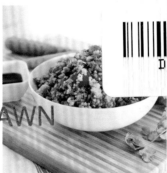

THE
Low-FODMAP IBS Solution
PLAN & COOKBOOK

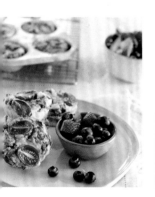
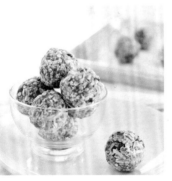
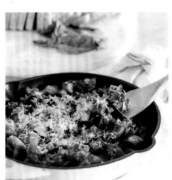
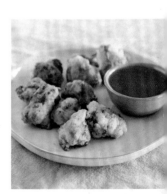

"Rachel Pauls, M.D., has leveraged her experiences as a physician, patient, and entrepreneur to create a tour de force which will help persons with digestive issues better understand the why, how, and how long of the low-FODMAP diet plan. I will be adding *The Low-FODMAP IBS Solution Plan and Cookbook* to my patients' reading list."

— **William D. Chey, M.D., Nostrant Collegiate Professor of Gastroenterology and Nutrition Sciences Director, Digestive Disorders Nutrition & Behavioral Health Program, University of Michigan Health System**

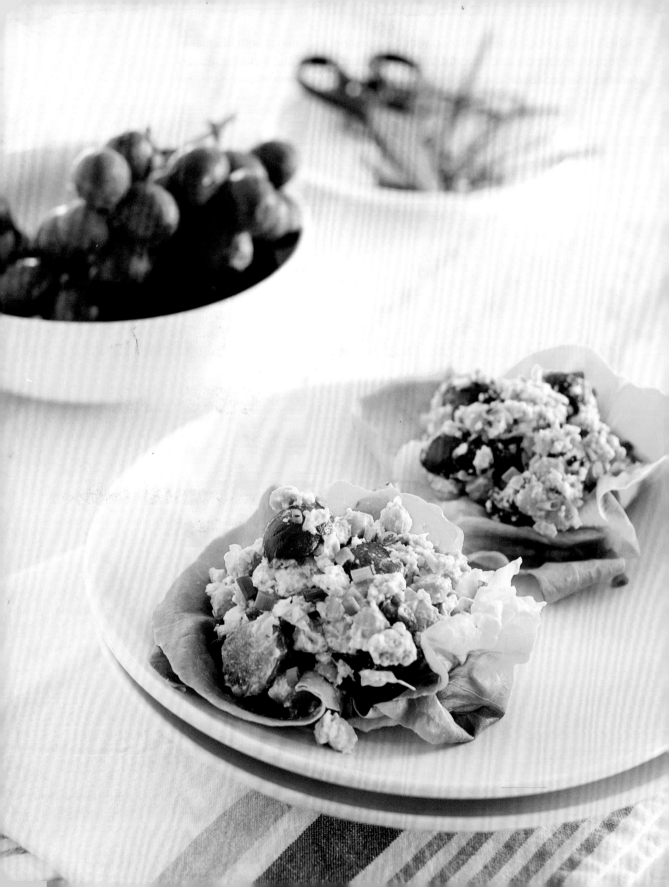

THE
Low-FODMAP
IBS Solution
PLAN & COOKBOOK

Heal Your IBS with More Than 100 Low-FODMAP Recipes That Prep in 30 Minutes or Less

Rachel Pauls, M.D.

FAIR WINDS

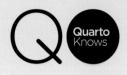

Inspiring | Educating | Creating | Entertaining

Brimming with creative inspiration, how-to projects, and useful information to enrich your everyday life, Quarto Knows is a favorite destination for those pursuing their interests and passions. Visit our site and dig deeper with our books into your area of interest: Quarto Creates, Quarto Cooks, Quarto Homes, Quarto Lives, Quarto Drives, Quarto Explores, Quarto Gifts, or Quarto Kids.

First Published in 2020 by Fair Winds Press, an imprint of The Quarto Group,
100 Cummings Center, Suite 265-D, Beverly, MA 01915, USA.
T (978) 282-9590 F (978) 283-2742 QuartoKnows.com

Fair Winds Press titles are also available at discount for retail, wholesale, promotional, and bulk purchase. For details, contact the Special Sales Manager by email at specialsales@quarto.com or by mail at The Quarto Group, Attn: Special Sales Manager, 100 Cummings Center, Suite 265-D, Beverly, MA 01915, USA.

24 23 22 21 20   1 2 3 4 5

ISBN: 978-1-59233-971-6

Digital edition published in 2020
eISBN: 978-1-63159-910-1

Library of Congress Cataloging-in-Publication Data

Pauls, Rachel, author.

The low-FODMAP IBS solution plan and cookbook: heal your IBS with more than 100 low-FODMAP recipes that prep in 30 minutes or less /

Rachel Pauls, M.D.

ISBN 9781592339716 (trade paperback) | ISBN 9781631599101 (ebook)

1. Irritable colon—Diet therapy—Recipes. 2. Irritable colon—Diet therapy. 3. Cookbooks.

RC862.I77 P38 2020 | 641.5/631—dc23

2020011585

Design: Amy Sly

Photography: Alison Bickel

Illustration: Rachel Pauls Food

Printed in China

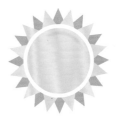

IMPORTANT NOTE FROM THE AUTHOR

This book should not be relied upon for any medical or dietary advice or replace the care of a health care provider. The research and science surrounding FODMAPs and IBS is rapidly evolving. While the recipes in this book are intended to be low-FODMAP based upon available information at the time of writing (2020), none of them has been subjected to formal laboratory analysis for FODMAPs. If you experience negative symptoms related to any of the recipes, stop eating that food and contact your health care provider.

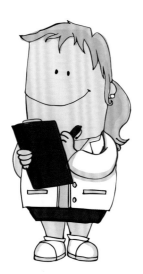

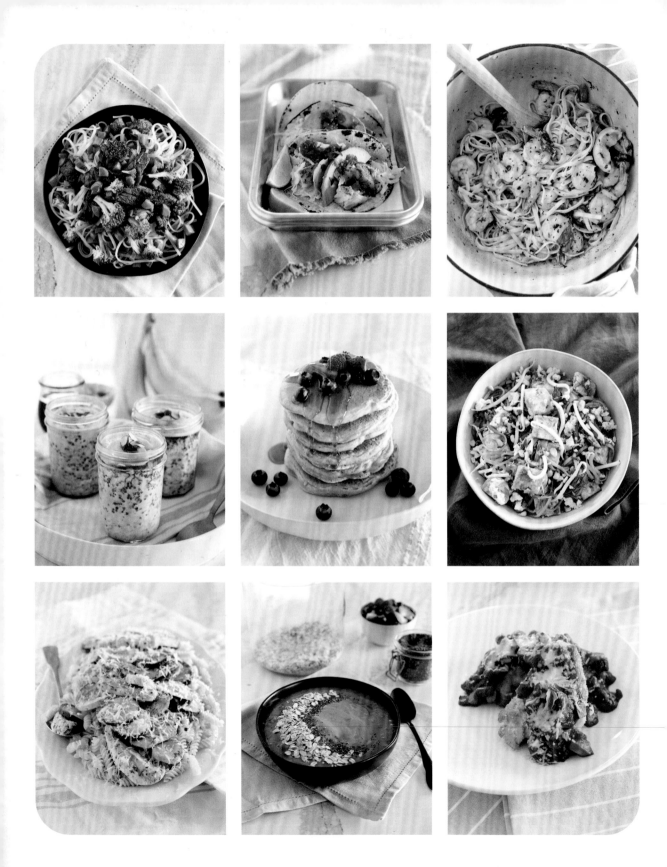

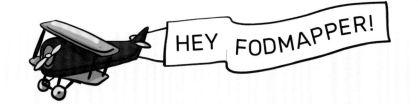

CONTENTS

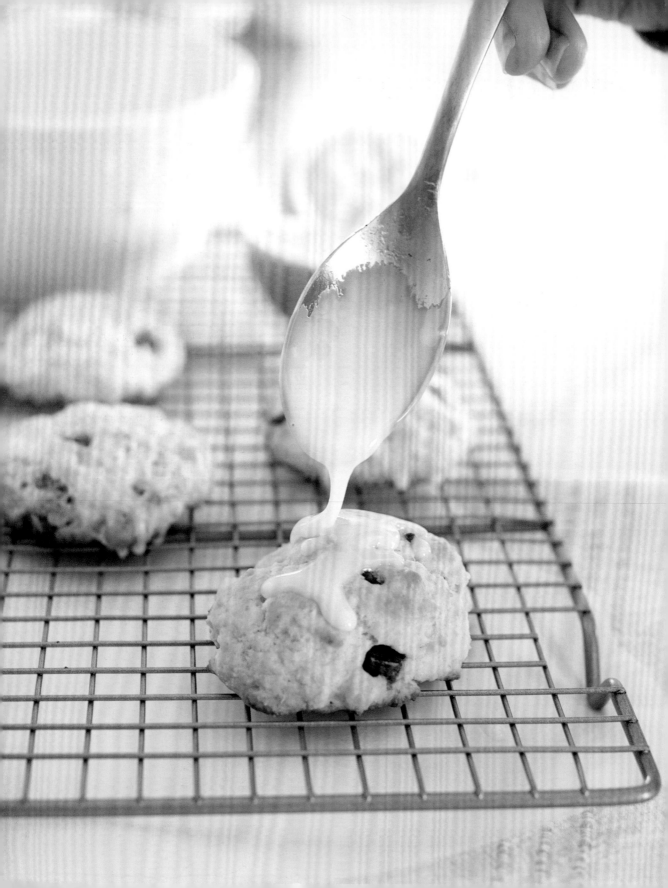

INTRODUCTION

Welcome!

I am so glad to meet you.

We are going to be embarking on an exciting journey. A journey that will change your life.

If you are reading this book, chances are that you have irritable bowel syndrome (IBS) or another digestive problem. The symptoms are intrusive and impacting your life. You are here because you need help.

You have come to the right place. I am going to provide you with the *solution* for your digestive problems. This solution will heal your gut, balance your spirit, and result in a healthier and happier you.

A healthy intestine is a very important aspect of our overall well-being. In fact, up to 90 percent of our body's serotonin (our "happy hormone") is produced in our intestinal tract. That means that healing your gut can make you happy from the inside out. A healthy intestine has also been linked with better immunity, greater energy, and sharper focus. Don't those sound amazing?

Healing your IBS symptoms will lead to improvements in every part of your life. Would you like to sleep better? Take fewer sick days and achieve more success in your career? What about improving your comfort and spontaneity with intimacy?

You can have all those things. And more.

My solution to your IBS will not only make you feel healthier and happier, but it will empower you for the future.

How am I so certain? For starters, I have been a medical doctor for more than twenty years and have educated countless residents and fellows along the way. As a reconstructive pelvic surgeon who has operated on hundreds of women, I have intimate knowledge of the anatomy of the intestines and understand the role of that anatomy on bowel health. I have counseled patients about their gastrointestinal (GI) symptoms and am well aware of the role of diet in improving quality of life. I have published more than ninety-five academic articles and know the ins and outs of all the research.

But that is not the main reason I can help you.

The main reason is, I am just like you. I have IBS. And I have been there. Wearing loose clothes so that my bloated belly wouldn't hurt as the day went on. Sleepless nights in and out of the bathroom. Wondering if I would ever figure out which foods were triggering my symptoms.

It all changed when I discovered the low-FODMAP diet.

The low-FODMAP diet healed me from the inside out. Changing my way of eating ignited my passion for cooking and baking, so I could enjoy my favorite meals without the triggering foods. I got my energy back, my mood improved, and a cloud lifted from my life. I truly became *happier*.

Now I am beginning a new adventure: sharing my expertise with you, through this book.

This book is for those of you with IBS who are like me. Real people living in the real world. In this book, you will receive all the knowledge and skills to begin the low-FODMAP diet. I'll explain the *why*, the *how*, and the *when*. I will provide you with a four-week meal plan to keep you on track. I will give you shopping lists, ways to manage social situations, and loads of other information.

I'll share 104 of my favorite, delicious recipes plus eleven bonus recipes that come together in 30 minutes or less. All are gluten-free, and many are allergy-friendly, vegan, or vegetarian. After those four weeks of success, I won't abandon you. I will teach you the next steps so that you can continue to feel your best. This book has everything you need.

Are you ready to heal your IBS symptoms, improve your energy, and embark on the path to a healthier and happier you?

This is our journey.

Let's do it.

Rachel Pauls, M.D.

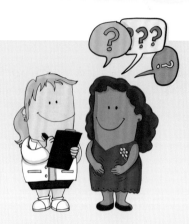

IRRITABLE BOWEL SYNDROME (IBS) AND THE IBS SOLUTION

Are you ready to get started with the solution to your irritable bowel syndrome (IBS) and digestive problems?

+ In the first chapter of this book, I will cover everything you need to know about IBS. I will review the symptoms, triggers, and available treatments, including the low-FODMAP diet.

+ You will learn how to set up your home for the low-FODMAP diet in order to be most successful. I will help you with your grocery list and show you all my secrets.

+ Then, you will receive your four-week meal plan, which will provide guidance each and every day toward a healthier and happier you.

+ Finally, I will teach you about 'reintroduction and personalization', which will be the key to your IBS solution forever.

IRRITABLE BOWEL SYNDROME: WHAT, WHY, AND HOW TO

Irritable bowel syndrome, or IBS, is the most common "functional" gastrointestinal (GI, or gut) disorder in the world.

A "functional" GI disorder is a disorder of the digestive system that results from a problem in the function, or behavior, of the intestines, rather than the actual structure, anatomy, or chemistry. That means it isn't related to cancer, celiac disease, or ulcerative colitis. But it is related to chronic (or relapsing/recurring) symptoms, which result in a negative impact on the quality of life of the person with the condition.

About 10 percent of people worldwide have IBS (which is a huge number), but it may actually be a lot more. We think that people tend to live with symptoms for years before discussing them with their doctor.

IBS has a massive impact on our society. It has been documented as the second most frequent reason for missing work (following the common cold) and is responsible for enormous costs to our medical system.

Researchers believe IBS results from a combination of:

- **Altered** movement of the intestine,

- **Enhanced** sensation of the movement in that individual, and

- **Disorganized** signals between the gut and the brain.

 Essentially, there is a difference in not only *what happens* in the gut of people with IBS but also in the way they *experience* those differences.

Let's look at the classic example of chili and beans. Eating chili and beans causes gas and bloating, to some degree, in almost everyone. However, when someone *without IBS* eats chili, they may or may not feel uncomfortable with the gas and bloating. Compare that to a person *with IBS* eating the same chili and beans. The symptoms they have may be so profound that they need to take a day or two off work.

Unfortunately, medical research hasn't discovered what causes IBS.

Since we don't know exactly *why* it happens, there is no "cure." That's the bad news.

But there is good news too. We have come a long way toward understanding the common triggers for IBS. This means that we have many ways to help keep the symptoms *under control.*

One of the best ways to improve IBS is to eliminate the parts of your life that may be "triggers." A trigger is something that can stimulate IBS symptoms by irritating your intestine in a particular way. Because your intestine is more sensitive (due to your IBS), these triggers are more likely to cause symptoms. Here are some common IBS triggers:

- **Food:** This is the number one trigger for IBS symptoms, but you knew that, didn't you? Studies show that people with IBS *know* that what they eat leads to their symptoms. The challenge is figuring out what those foods are. That is how this book is going to help you.

  + **FODMAPs:** *FODMAP* is an acronym for fermentable oligo-, di-, monosaccharides and polyols (we'll be looking more at what this acronym means later in the chapter). These are carbohydrates that can be a trigger for many of the symptoms that people with IBS find most uncomfortable. Thus, eliminating high-FODMAP foods is the most effective dietary treatment for IBS and is the basis of the changes you will make.

  + **Gluten:** Many people with IBS find gluten causes worsening GI symptoms. This is independent of celiac disease and is called non-celiac gluten sensitivity.

  + **Dairy:** Lactose is a high-FODMAP food and is poorly digested by many people with IBS.

- **Carbonation:** Drinks with carbonation irritate the intestines and may stimulate symptoms of IBS.

- **Spicy foods:** Highly spiced foods may cause both heartburn and IBS symptoms.

- **Alcohol:** Alcohol is a gut irritant and can lead to both diarrhea and constipation.

- **Fiber:** While many of us have been told to eat more fiber, it isn't *always* the cure for our symptoms, and some types are better than others (we will discuss fiber again later in this chapter).

- **Fatty and greasy foods:** These can lead to increased movement in the gut and diarrhea as well as cramping.

- **Excess sugar:** High amounts of sugar can be difficult on the digestion and lead to IBS symptoms.

- **Stress:** Recent research has established several connections between our brains and our gut. Although stress and anxiety don't directly *cause* IBS (it isn't in your head), they can lead to our bodies being less able to manage the symptoms and therefore trigger episodes. I will provide you with several strategies to manage stress at the end of this chapter.

- **Inadequate sleep:** Sleep is critical to feeling happy and energized. Most of us don't get nearly enough rest, which can translate into a diminished immune system and increase likelihood of IBS flare-ups. We will review important sleeping tips on page 17. Keep reading!

- **Smoking:** Tobacco is an irritant to the GI tract, so smoking can lead to worse symptoms of IBS.

- **Pelvic floor dysfunction:** Dysfunction of the pelvic supports (prolapse) can result in difficulty evacuating bowel movements and worsen constipation. If you suspect a problem in this area, then seek out a specialist in female pelvic medicine and reconstructive surgery (my subspecialty).

This book will show you how to manage all these triggers of IBS. I will share my four-week meal plan and easy recipes that will limit the food triggers you see above. I will also give you tips to manage stress, improve your sleep, and enhance your mind-body connection. The results will be astounding. You will sleep better, have more energy, and feel healthier and happier. Let's continue learning!

COMMON SYMPTOMS OF IBS

Here are some of the common IBS symptoms. You don't need to have *all* of these to be diagnosed with IBS.

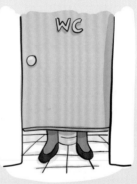

- Abdominal pain, cramping

- Constipation

- Diarrhea

- Alternating constipation and diarrhea

- Change in the way stool looks (may be harder or softer, may contain mucus)

- Excess or painful gas, bloating

- Symptoms related to meals or certain foods

- Difficulty sleeping

- Mood disturbance, such as depression

HOW IS IBS DIAGNOSED?

Doctors often discuss and describe IBS based on something called the "Rome Diagnostic Criteria." What exactly are those?

Well, a panel of doctors and experts in treating IBS came together (in Rome, Italy) in 1988. The panel met to create guidelines to establish whether someone has IBS. These guidelines became known as the "Rome Criteria."

As our understanding of IBS has changed, the Rome Criteria have been modified. The latest version of the guidelines is called the "Rome IV Criteria for IBS" (2016). (See sidebar below.)

So *that* is the main way doctors diagnose IBS—by using the symptoms below. In other words, there is not any physical exam finding, blood test, X-ray, computerized tomography (CT) scan, or magnetic resonance imaging (MRI) scan that diagnoses IBS. A doctor can't put a scope in your intestine to "see" IBS or find it on a biopsy. A stool specimen cannot tell whether you have it.

However, it's possible that your doctor will order some of the above medical tests. This could be important to confirm that you don't have *another* diagnosis. For example, some other possible causes for symptoms similar to IBS are inflammatory bowel disease (Crohn's disease and ulcerative colitis), celiac disease (gluten intolerance), diverticulitis, acid reflux (GERD), lactose intolerance, food allergies, gastroparesis, small intestinal bacterial overgrowth (SIBO), pelvic organ prolapse, or colon cancer.

WHY YOU? WHY NOW?

I often get asked "why" by my patients. Why did this happen to them? Did something cause it? Why now?

Typically, it is difficult to pinpoint a cause. Because IBS is caused by disruptions in the way food is digested, as well as how those disruptions are perceived, multiple factors are involved.

However, one of the interesting factors that has recently received a lot of attention is the *intestinal microbiome*. The microbiome is the unique array of bacteria found naturally in our bodies. These bacteria "colonize" our organs, but don't cause us harm (this is different from the types of bacteria that cause infections or for which we take antibiotics). Our intestines have a special and unique microbiome, and the microbiome differs from person to person. Because your microbiome depends on your diet to a large degree, it will change depending on where (and when) you live.

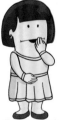

ROME IV CRITERIA FOR IBS

Recurrent abdominal pain at least one day per week in the last three months (on average) in association with two or more of the following:

- Defecation, or having a bowel movement (which could either increase or decrease the pain)
- A change in stool frequency
- A change in stool form (or appearance)

TALKING TO YOUR DOCTOR

Here are some questions to ask your doctor if you suspect you have IBS:

- Could some other condition be causing my symptoms? Could I have inflammatory bowel disease or celiac disease, for example?

- Should I be following a certain diet? If so, what diet do you suggest?

- Do you have a dietitian or nutritionist you would recommend that I work with?

- Would medications help my symptoms? If so, what are possible side effects of the medications and how would they work?

- Do you recommend any other treatments, such as supplements, probiotics, or holistic approaches (acupuncture, yoga), for my IBS?

Signs of a more serious condition include blood in the stool, anemia, weight loss, a narrowed appearance to bowel movements, weakness, feeling like you haven't completely evacuated after a bowel movement, swelling or rash, fever or nausea/vomiting, symptoms that wake you in the middle of the night, and a family history of colon cancer or inflammatory bowel disease.

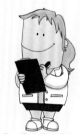

Research has suggested that the intestinal microbiome may be a key to unlocking some of the mysteries and treatments of IBS. While knowledge is evolving, we know that the foods we eat cause subtle changes in our microbiome. These changes impact intestinal symptoms. In other words, dietary changes create intestinal changes that could lead to improved symptoms.

MANAGING IBS: WE ARE WHAT WE EAT

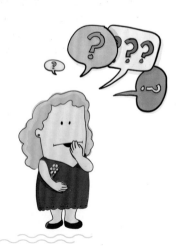

Studies have shown that *all* individuals (with or without IBS) perceive that certain foods trigger their GI symptoms. However, people with IBS are *more likely* to restrict food and avoid *more types* of food than people without IBS. It makes sense. What we eat and drink enters our stomach, then our intestines. If that food or beverage is difficult to digest, it is more likely to trigger symptoms of gas, bloating, diarrhea, or constipation.

- Unsurprisingly, over the years, researchers have attempted to find the best eating plan to help patients with IBS. To date, the single most effective one is the low-FODMAP diet.

- In fact, dozens of studies over the past decade have proven that a low-FODMAP diet improves symptoms of IBS in 70 to 80 percent of patients. That is better than medications (without the high costs and side effects)!

- The low-FODMAP diet has been shown to improve symptoms in other GI conditions besides IBS, such as Crohn's, colitis, and SIBO.

- Furthermore, the low-FODMAP diet is a wonderful stepping-stone to learn which foods may be triggers for you. This helps guide your future "modified low-FODMAP" lifestyle (discussed on page 31).

- For all these reasons, I believe strongly that the low-FODMAP diet is the best initial approach for IBS symptoms.

By this point, you have gotten an idea about how helpful the low-FODMAP diet is. But you still don't know what it means to follow a low-FODMAP diet. That's our next topic!

THE LOW-FODMAP DIET: FOD-WHAT?

The low-FODMAP diet was introduced in Australia in the early 2000s. A group of doctors and researchers studying IBS recognized the impact that carbohydrates have on GI symptoms. They sought to classify carbohydrates based on whether they were more or less likely to cause GI symptoms. This is what "FODMAP" stands for:

F: Fermentable (can be broken down by bacteria in the intestine and made into gas)

O: Oligosaccharides (carbohydrates made up of chains of sugars, such as onion, inulin, and beans)

D: Disaccharides (carbohydrates made of two linked sugars, such as lactose in dairy products)

M: Monosaccharides (carbohydrates made of one sugar, such as fructose found in apples and honey)

A: And

P: Poylalcohols (examples include sorbitol, maltitol in sugar-free gums and mints, and certain medications)

WHY A LOW-FODMAP DIET WORKS

Let me explain a bit more. Carbohydrates are in almost everything we eat, even foods without calories (like artificial sweeteners and tea). Some of those carbohydrates are harder to digest. Since your intestine doesn't break them down easily, they may create more water movement in the gut (causing diarrhea). They also linger for more time in the colon, allowing bacteria to ferment them (causing gas). As a result of the imbalance in water movement, these carbohydrates can also be associated with constipation. Basically, these are the symptoms of IBS.

Some foods have high levels of the poorly digestible FODMAPs (high-FODMAP food) and some have low or no FODMAPs (low-FODMAP food). By avoiding the high-FODMAP foods, you can reduce the symptoms associated with them.

The advantage of the low-FODMAP diet is it eliminates all these noxious foods and beverages for four to six weeks in order to allow your gut to heal and to balance out your system. That is the first step. It is known as the *elimination phase*. This book is meant to guide you through the first four weeks of the elimination phase, to heal your gut and give

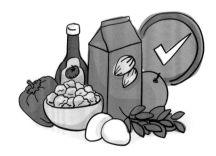

you the solution for your IBS. During the elimination phase, it will be important to follow the low-FODMAP diet exclusively in order to ensure your success.

After the first four weeks of the elimination phase, you may be ready to try reintroducing foods one at a time. The advantage of starting with the elimination phase is that it provides you with a stable, clean gut. That makes it much easier to identify which foods are triggers for you. This second phase of the diet is known as *reintroduction and personalization*, and I will guide you through this stage as well. Once you are finished with the personalization phase, you will likely be following a "personalized" or "modified" low-FODMAP diet. That will be the solution to your IBS forever.

TIPS FOR LOW-FODMAP EATING

Here are a few important concepts:

- There is no such thing as a "no-FODMAP diet." As long as you stick to foods that are lower in FODMAPs, you should be able to avoid symptoms.

- Low-FODMAP does not equal gluten-free. Gluten is a protein, and FODMAPs are carbohydrates. That being said, wheat and barley are high-FODMAP foods. As a result, I recommend gluten-free products as a part of the low-FODMAP diet, provided those products don't contain other high-FODMAP additives.

- Low-FODMAP does not mean dairy-free. You can have foods that are low in lactose but still contain dairy (such as some cheeses or lactose-free milks).

- Portion size matters. If something is low-FODMAP, you can have it as long as you pay attention to how much and don't have *more* than one low-FODMAP serving at a time. For example, you can have 10 almonds on the low-FODMAP diet, but if you eat more than that (at the same time), then you will end up with a high-FODMAP portion.

- The low-FODMAP diet is not a "diet" to lose weight. The goal is to control your IBS symptoms and make you feel better, inside and out. The low-FODMAP recipes in this book are meant to taste delicious, so you don't feel deprived. It is tough enough as it is!

- While alcohol is allowed on the low-FODMAP diet, be aware that it is still a gut irritant. I recommend avoiding alcohol during the elimination phase of the low-FODMAP diet.

- Similarly, spicy foods, carbonation, and excessive fat or sugar can be tough to digest for many. Watch out for those items if you know they are triggers for you.

- In general, information regarding FODMAP levels have been provided by the scientists and doctors who designed the diet. They are based at Monash

STACKING

FODMAPs may accumulate in your intestine during a given day (this is known as "stacking"). Thus, it isn't always the food that you just ate causing your symptoms but may be the snack you ate earlier that has made its way to your intestine. This is one of the reasons it can be tricky to know which foods are the triggers for your IBS.

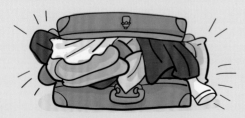

Imagine your intestines are a suitcase that you are packing with clothes (food). At first, the suitcase is comfortable and light. But as you continue to pack it with clothes, it becomes more and more distended. That is what happens in your gut over the course of the day if you eat foods that are not easily digested.

University in Australia. The information is shared via the Monash app (see sidebar on page 18). The recommended serving size is listed for all of the foods to help you know how much to enjoy.

OTHER IBS TREATMENTS

While the low-FODMAP diet is an incredibly important part of your IBS solution, sometimes it isn't enough. I will review other IBS treatments that may be useful, so that you can improve your chance for success.

STRESS MANAGEMENT

One of the most beneficial ways to improve your health is to reduce the impact of stress. While you can't eliminate stressful events from your life, you can become more equipped to deal with them.

Here are strategies to manage stress that I personally practice, as well as recommend to my patients:

- **Meditation and mindfulness:** Practicing mindfulness while eating, and in all aspects of your life, encourages contentment and balance. Put away your cell phone during meals!

- **Yoga:** There are specific yoga poses designed to help IBS that are simple to learn. See my website at www.rachelpaulsfood.com/five-amazing-yoga-poses-help-reduce-ibs-symptoms.

- **Acupuncture:** Several studies have shown acupuncture to have a beneficial impact on IBS.

- **Exercise:** Exercise is a wonderful way to reduce your stress and improve your IBS symptoms.

- **Sleep hygiene:** Getting at least eight hours of sleep each night has been shown to decrease all sorts of medical issues, not just IBS. Some ways to work on your sleep hygiene include:

  + Go to bed and wake up at the same time each day.

  + Keep your room dark at night (turn off the TV).

  + Exercise during the day.

  + Avoid caffeine or nicotine closer to bedtime.

  + Avoid large meals before bedtime.

  + Set up a comfortable sleep environment (pillows, room temperature).

PROBIOTICS

Several studies suggest that probiotics reduce symptoms of IBS. They also seem to work well in conjunction with the low-FODMAP diet. I think it's reasonable to try a probiotic supplement to see if it helps, but it does not replace other dietary interventions.

FIBER

While fiber isn't always the answer to everyone's symptoms, psyllium fiber may be useful in treating constipation associated with IBS.

COUNSELING AND MENTAL HEALTH SUPPORT

If you are struggling with your mood and wonder whether you could have depression or anxiety, then reach out to your doctor. Untreated mental health issues will contribute to IBS symptoms.

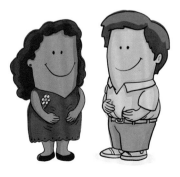

HOW TO READ LABELS

In general, I recommend eating whole foods while on the low-FODMAP diet. Not only do unprocessed foods taste better (in my opinion), but they are also more likely to be healthy for you. Plus, you can be certain what is in the product and thereby ensure you interpret correctly your body's reaction to it.

Nevertheless, eating prepared food is a necessary part of our lives. Having basic knowledge about reading ingredient lists on food labels is the key to interpreting whether something is safe for you to enjoy. The caveat is that you must *always* read food labels. With today's food sensitivity awareness, it is not unusual to make a request about ingredients. Don't be embarrassed!

When reading a label, it is important to understand that all ingredients are listed in order of *weight*. So, the item listed first has the highest weight in the product, and the last item may be only a tiny fraction of the product. You may still be able to tolerate the food if the high-FODMAP additive is the last listed ingredient. See my website (www.rachelpaulsfood.com/how-to-read-labels/) for a list of high-FODMAP foods that you should look out for on labels.

THE MONASH APP

I highly recommend purchasing the Monash app for your mobile device. It has the most comprehensive list of high- and low-FODMAP foods and is updated regularly.

You can also find free downloadable lists of high- and low-FODMAP foods and food additives at www.rachelpaulsfood.com and www.katescarlata.com.

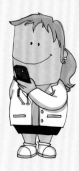

LAYING THE FOUNDATION FOR YOUR SUCCESS

CULTIVATE YOUR ENVIRONMENT: SET UP A SUPPORT NETWORK

The first step in beginning any successful lifestyle change is to set up a support network. Be *proactive*, not *reactive*, to limit awkward situations and temptations.

Share your plans with family and close friends, and make them aware you are beginning a new dietary plan to treat your IBS symptoms. Let them know what to expect in the coming weeks. You never know: They may decide to participate with you!

Next, you will want to set up your kitchen with the right equipment to help maximize your meal plan.

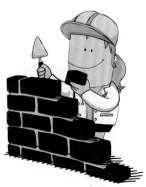

PREPARE YOUR KITCHEN: TOOLS AND EQUIPMENT

Here are the kitchen tools and equipment that will help you be successful on the low-FODMAP diet:

- **Kitchen scale:** You will need this item to verify suitable low-FODMAP portion sizes. Since Monash University is based in Australia, their low-FODMAP app delineates portion size based on weight (often in grams). This will be the most accurate method to determine a safe amount to eat.

- **Measuring cups and measuring spoons:** Note that dry items (like flour) need to be measured with a dry measuring cup, and liquids (like oil) go in a liquid measuring cup. They are not equivalent.

- **Citrus fruit juicer:** You will find your juicer invaluable for squeezing fresh lemons, limes, and oranges for recipes (I have a little handheld one). Do not substitute processed juices, as those tend to be high-FODMAP.

- **Fruit zester:** Using the zest from lemons, limes, and oranges will give a recipe amazing flavor. The zest contains the oils from the fruit and is very potent.

- **Blender:** This is invaluable for making smoothies.

- **Immersion blender:** These handheld blenders on a stick are nice for blending salad dressings, soups, and sauces.

- **Storage containers of various sizes:** Storage containers will streamline your weekly meal plan. I like glass containers for eating at home and microwave-safe plastic for packing lunches.

- **Mason jars:** Small jars are very useful for mixing dressings, dips, overnight oats, and chia pudding and for pickling vegetables.

- **Parchment paper:** This is very useful for baking. Baking without gluten can be sticky, and parchment paper makes removal from pans a dream.

GIVE YOUR PANTRY A MAKEOVER

I recommend clearing out your pantry and fridge to reduce the chances of temptation or mistakes. Here are ways to begin:

- Remove onion or garlic from your refrigerator and spice racks. Note that "natural flavoring" in savory products typically contains onion and/or garlic.

- Eliminate any condiments, sauces, and snack foods with high-fructose corn syrup, fructose, honey, molasses, or agave.

- Give away any energy bars or processed foods with inulin, chicory root, or FOS (fructooligosaccharides). Make sure your coffee doesn't contain chicory (some dark-roasted blends do).

- Check your vitamins and supplements for sorbitol additives and ditch your sugar-free gum or mints.

- Screen foods touted as "high fiber," as they may contain high-FODMAP additives like inulin or FOS.

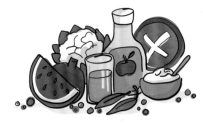

LOW-FODMAP INGREDIENT SUBSTITUTIONS

One of the concerns many people have when beginning the low-FODMAP diet is that they won't be able to enjoy foods with flavor or their favorite recipes. This is untrue. Here are my simple ingredient substitutions that won't sacrifice your palate or your tummy.

High-FODMAP Ingredient	Substitution
AGAVE	Light corn syrup, maple syrup
BREADCRUMBS	Gluten-free low-FODMAP breadcrumbs, or make your own using your choice of low-FODMAP bread
CANNED CORN	Fresh frozen corn or freshly made corn on the cob with kernels removed
COUSCOUS	Quinoa or rice
FLOUR (wheat based)	Gluten-free rice or corn-based flours with low-FODMAP ingredients; avoid almond flour, coconut flour, and those with chickpeas, peas, or beans in their blends Xanthan gum, a powder that will need to be added to your gluten-free flour if it isn't already; it helps with gluten-free baking texture
HEAVY CREAM	Canned coconut cream
HONEY	Light corn syrup, maple syrup
MILK	Lactose-free milk, almond milk, hemp milk
MOLASSES	Dark corn syrup or maple syrup
ONION AND GARLIC (check spice blends, chips, nuts, crackers, stocks, sauces, and canned vegetables)	Oils infused with garlic, onion, or shallot* Asafoetida, a spice that imparts onion or garlic flavor Chives, green scallion tips
PASTA (wheat based)	Gluten-free pastas with low-FODMAP ingredients (rice, corn based)
PROTEIN POWDER WITH WHEY, INULIN, OR OTHER HIGH-FODMAP INGREDIENTS	Brown rice protein powders, protein powders using whey protein isolate (lower in lactose levels)
SOUP BASES, MARINADES, CONDIMENTS, AND SAUCES WITH ONION AND GARLIC	Prepared soup bases, spice blends, and marinades from low-FODMAP food vendors**, or make your own with the recipes in chapter 8
SPAGHETTI SAUCE (jar)	Spaghetti sauce without onion or garlic**, or use my recipe on page 116 to make your own

* FODMAPs are soluble (dissolve) in water, but not in oil. That means if you cook onion in a broth, then remove the onion pieces, the onion's FODMAPs have already leached into the liquid. Don't eat it! However, if you use onion-infused olive oil, then you will have the onion flavor, but not the stomachache.

** See notes opposite, as well as the grocery shopping section for tips on my preferred brands for these ingredients.

Some of the ingredients above are not always easy to find at standard grocery stores. However, there are online stores that sell certified low-FODMAP foods.

Certified low-FODMAP means they have undergone laboratory testing verifying them to be low-FODMAP. Here are a few brands to consider; you may have others in your area too.

Rachel Pauls Food: Low-FODMAP energy bars, beef jerky, spice blends, soup bases, and baking mixes

FODY Foods: Low-FODMAP spaghetti sauces, marinades, condiments, salad dressings, infused olive oils, soup bases, spice blends, and energy bars

Casa de Sante: Low-FODMAP simmer sauces, spice blends, condiments, and protein powders

HELPFUL HINTS

Here are some tips that will help make the transition to a low-FODMAP diet easier:

- **Get ready before you shop.** Your first shopping trip may seem overwhelming. Here's how to prepare:

  + Plan your menus for the week before you shop (I will help you with the grocery list below).

  + Bring a high/low-FODMAP food list or download the Monash app to your mobile device.

  + Designate less busy times for your grocery shopping or order online first.

- **Allocate time for food prep.** Make some of your breakfasts or lunches for the week, and put them in ready-to-go containers. Many of my low-FODMAP recipes have tips for making ahead.

- **Your freezer is your friend.** If I am making a low-FODMAP casserole recipe, I double or triple it and then freeze the other servings in a resealable freezer bag or covered dish. That way, I have something ready to go in a week or two!

- **Stock the right snacks at home and work.** Having your favorite snacks that are also low-FODMAP in your kitchen, gym bag, and desk at work will mean less chance you will reach for something high-FODMAP when the cravings strike.

- **Know your options for eating out.** Plan ahead. If eating at a friend's, bring a low-FODMAP dish to share. If dining out, call ahead to verify they have options for you.

- **Travel smart.** Don't forget to pack some low-FODMAP fuel in your carry-on.

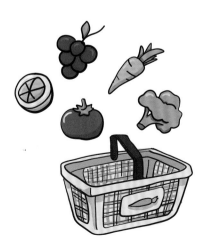

THE BIG SHOPPING SPREE

Now we are ready to go grocery shopping, armed with our low-FODMAP grocery shopping list. Don't worry—I will make it easy!

If you are following the four-week meal plan, use this list as your guide. Perishable items you will be using for the first week of the meal plan are starred with one asterisk (*). Nonperishable items that you will need for the four-week meal plan have two asterisks (**) next to them.

LOW-FODMAP GROCERY SHOPPING LIST

FRESH FRUITS

- ☐ Bananas*
- ☐ Blueberries*
- ☐ Cantaloupe
- ☐ Grapes*
- ☐ Kiwi
- ☐ Lemons*
- ☐ Limes*
- ☐ Oranges*
- ☐ Pineapple
- ☐ Raspberries
- ☐ Strawberries*
- ☐ Tomatoes
  Cherry tomatoes*, standard tomatoes*

FRESH VEGETABLES

- ☐ Bean sprouts
- ☐ Broccoli* (heads only)
- ☐ Cabbage
- ☐ Carrots*
- ☐ Celery* (you will need only one stalk for the recipe)
- ☐ Chile peppers
- ☐ Collard greens
- ☐ Corn** (fresh or fresh frozen)

- ☐ Cucumbers*
- ☐ Eggplant
- ☐ Green beans
- ☐ Green bell peppers
- ☐ Kale
- ☐ Lettuce*
  Arugula, butter/Bibb*, iceberg, romaine
- ☐ Parsnips**
- ☐ Potatoes*
  New potatoes*, russet potatoes*, shredded potatoes**
- ☐ Red bell peppers*
- ☐ Scallions (green tips only)
- ☐ Spaghetti squash
- ☐ Spinach*
- ☐ Sweet potatoes
- ☐ Yams
- ☐ Yellow squash
- ☐ Zucchini*

FRESH HERBS

- ☐ Basil*
- ☐ Chives*
- ☐ Dill*
- ☐ Ginger root*
- ☐ Parsley*
- ☐ Rosemary*

CANNED OR JARRED FRUITS AND VEGETABLES

- ☐ Artichoke hearts*
- ☐ Baby corn
- ☐ Bamboo shoots**
- ☐ Capers**
- ☐ Chickpeas**
- ☐ Hearts of palm**
- ☐ Lentils*
- ☐ Olives
  Black, green**, kalamata**

- ☐ **Pure pumpkin***
- ☐ **Tomatoes**

  Diced tomatoes*, pureed tomatoes*, tomato paste*

  Make sure no added spices

  You will need all three of these for the first week of the meal plan
- ☐ **Water chestnuts****

DRIED HERBS AND SPICES (ENSURE NO ONION/GARLIC ADDED TO SPICE BLENDS)

- ☐ **Allspice**
- ☐ **Ancho chile**
- ☐ **Basil**
- ☐ **Bay leaves***
- ☐ **Black peppercorns with grinder***
- ☐ **Cardamom**
- ☐ **Cayenne pepper****
- ☐ **Chives****
- ☐ **Cilantro**
- ☐ **Cinnamon***
- ☐ **Cloves**
- ☐ **Coriander****
- ☐ **Cream of tartar**
- ☐ **Cumin****
- ☐ **Dill**
- ☐ **Garam masala**
- ☐ **Ginger****
- ☐ **Marjoram**
- ☐ **Mustard powder****
- ☐ **Nutmeg****
- ☐ **Oregano****

- ☐ **Paprika****
- ☐ **Parsley****
- ☐ **Pumpkin pie spice***
- ☐ **Red pepper flakes****
- ☐ **Rosemary****
- ☐ **Sage**
- ☐ **Sea salt***
- ☐ **Spice blends***

  Italian blended seasoning*, taco seasoning*, steak seasoning

  See page 21 for suggestions on low-FODMAP vendors for spice blends
- ☐ **Stock/soup mixes* (powder or paste)**

  Vegetable**, chicken**, beef

  See page 21 for online low-FODMAP stock vendors
- ☐ **Thyme****
- ☐ **Turmeric**
- ☐ **Yellow curry****

DAIRY

- ☐ **Butter or vegan margarine***

  Check ingredients and avoid vegan margarine with cashews
- ☐ **Cheese**

  Cheddar*, mozzarella*, mozzarella sticks*, Colby Jack, Brie, Parmesan, feta, Swiss, goat

  Be wary of "shredded cheese blends," as they sometimes contain onion and/or garlic
- ☐ **Lactose-free cream cheese or regular cream cheese (2 tablespoons [30 g] per serving)**

- ☐ **Lactose-free sour cream or regular sour cream (2 tablespoons [30 g] per serving)**
- ☐ **Lactose-free yogurt or coconut yogurt for vegan***

  Green Valley Organics is a low-FODMAP certified brand for lactose-free dairy products
- ☐ **Milk of choice**

  Lactose-free milk*, unsweetened almond milk*, hemp milk or rice milk for vegan

---

PROTEIN

- ☐ **Canned salmon (in water)**
- ☐ **Canned tuna* (in water)**
- ☐ **Chicken**

  Breasts*, thighs, whole chicken, chicken wings or thighs for making stock*
- ☐ **Deli smoked turkey* and ham* (plain)**
- ☐ **Eggs***
- ☐ **Fish**

  Tilapia, salmon*, cod, halibut, mahi-mahi
- ☐ **Ground beef* and steak***
- ☐ **Pork and bacon**
- ☐ **Shellfish**

  Scallops, shrimp, crab
- ☐ **Turkey and ground turkey**

VEGAN PROTEIN

- ☐ **Extra-firm or firm tofu****
- ☐ **Low-FODMAP protein powder***

  I like NutriBiotic vanilla-flavored brown rice protein powder

- ☐ **Nutritional yeast****
- ☐ **Tempeh**

  No onion/garlic or high-FODMAP additives

BREADS, PASTA, AND GRAINS

- ☐ **One or more low-FODMAP bread choices***

  I opt for Udi's gluten-free white sandwich bread, hamburger buns, and plain bagels (I like the hamburger buns the best, for everything). These are kept in the freezer section, usually in a gluten-free section.

  Schär has certified some of their gluten-free bread products as low-FODMAP

- ☐ **Gluten-free breadcrumbs with low-FODMAP ingredients***
- ☐ **Gluten-free pizza crust with low-FODMAP ingredients****

  Usually in the freezer section

  I like Udi's brand (does contain egg ingredients)

- ☐ **Corn tortillas or gluten-free flour tortillas with low-FODMAP ingredients****

  Sometimes the gluten-free tortillas are called "flatbreads"

  You can often substitute these for pizza crusts in cooking (good for a vegan option)

- ☐ **Gluten-free pastas with low-FODMAP ingredients***

  I like Ronzoni and Barilla brands

  You will use penne**, spaghetti*, spaghettini**, and macaroni** for the meal plan

- ☐ **Asian-style rice noodles****
- ☐ **Raw white quinoa* and quinoa flakes**
- ☐ **Rice**

  Brown, long-grain white*, basmati, Arborio, jasmine

  You will need long-grain white for the recipes; pick any others you enjoy

- ☐ **Cornmeal/polenta**

  I like Bob's Red Mill brand

- ☐ **Dried lentils****

CEREALS

- ☐ **Cornflake cereal****

  Check your brand to ensure it doesn't contain high-FODMAP additives such as honey or fruit concentrates

- ☐ **Plain packaged instant oatmeal**
- ☐ **Quick oats****
- ☐ **Rice crisp cereal**

  I like gluten-free Rice Krispies

- ☐ **Toasted O's cereal****

  I like Cheerios

- ☐ **Traditional old-fashioned rolled oats***

SNACKS

- ☐ **Corn chips (no added onion or garlic)**
- ☐ **Gluten-free cookies with low-FODMAP ingredients**

  I like Glutino chocolate creme and vanilla creme cookies

- ☐ **Gluten-free crackers with low-FODMAP ingredients***

  I like Glutino brand

  Schär's products are also certified low-FODMAP; check labels

- ☐ **Gluten-free pretzels with low-FODMAP ingredients***

  I like Snyder's brand

- ☐ **Popcorn****

  Plain prepared or unpopped kernels for you to make

- ☐ **Potato chips* (plain or plain ruffled)**
- ☐ **Rice cakes (plain)**

NUTS AND SEEDS

Note that dry-roasted nuts and seeds often contain onion and garlic.

- ☐ **Almonds****
- ☐ **Black poppyseeds****
- ☐ **Chia seeds***
- ☐ **Coconut, shredded (unsweetened* and sweetened**)**
- ☐ **Flaxseed meal***
- ☐ **Mixed nuts**

  Avoid cashews, pistachios, and large amounts of almonds

- ☐ **Peanuts (plain*, salted*)**
- ☐ **Pecans****
- ☐ **Pumpkin seeds****
- ☐ **Sesame seeds****
- ☐ **Sunflower seeds**
- ☐ **Walnuts***

BAKING SUPPLIES

- ☐ **Baking powder***
- ☐ **Baking soda****
- ☐ **Candy sprinkles/jimmies*** (for baking)
- ☐ **Cocoa powder****
- ☐ **Cooking spray* or vegetable shortening**
- ☐ **Corn syrup***
- ☐ **Cornstarch***
- ☐ **Dried cranberries****
- ☐ **Gluten-free all-purpose flour blend with low-FODMAP ingredients***

  I like King Arthur brand and Authentic Foods GF Classical Blend flours

  Lo-Fo Pantry sells low-FODMAP certified baking blends

- ☐ **Gluten-free all-purpose pancake/biscuit baking mix with low-FODMAP ingredients***

  I like gluten-free Bisquick Lo-Fo Pantry sells low-FODMAP certified baking blends

- ☐ **Oat flour****

  You can also process traditional rolled oats to create your own flour; see my tip on page 140

- ☐ **Pure vanilla extract***

- ☐ **Semisweet chocolate chips*** **and dark chocolate squares*** **for snacks**

  I like Enjoy Life brand low-FODMAP certified products

- ☐ **Stevia or sucralose**
- ☐ **Sugar**

  Brown sugar*, confectioners' sugar**, granulated sugar*

- ☐ **Xanthan gum***

  If your flour does not have this, you will need to add it for baking

---

CONDIMENTS

- ☐ **Canned coconut milk and coconut cream****
- ☐ **Hot sauce with low-FODMAP ingredients****

  I like Tabasco Original

- ☐ **Ketchup** (no high-fructose corn syrup)**
- ☐ **Marmalade**
- ☐ **Mayonnaise***

  There are three vegan mayo brands that appear low-FODMAP based on ingredients:
  JUST Mayo
  Best Foods Vegan
  Vegenaise

- ☐ **Mustard**

  Dijon*, yellow*

- ☐ **Nut and/or seed butter**

  Almond*, peanut**, sunflower seed* (if nut allergic)

  Packets of nut butter and sunflower seed butter are very convenient (Note: One low-FODMAP serving for peanut/sunflower seed butter is 2 tablespoons

[30 g], for almond butter it is 1 tablespoon [15 g])

- ☐ **Oils**

  Canola oil*, coconut oil (for a vegan option in baking**), olive oil*, toasted sesame oil**

  Infused olive oils: garlic*, onion**, other desired infused oil (Check specialty grocery stores or online vendors mentioned on page 21)

- ☐ **Pure maple syrup***
- ☐ **Pure strawberry jam (no high-fructose corn syrup)**
- ☐ **Spaghetti sauce without onion/garlic***

  I like Prego Sensitive Recipe, which is low-FODMAP certified, and Rao's Homemade Sensitive Formula brands

- ☐ **Tahini** (sesame seed paste)**
- ☐ **Tamari (gluten-free soy sauce) or regular soy sauce***
- ☐ **Vinegar**

  Apple cider*, balsamic, distilled white, red wine**, rice**

- ☐ **Worcestershire sauce**

BEVERAGES

- ☐ **Club soda**

  Limit carbonation during the elimination phase

- ☐ **Dry red wine, for cooking***

  Avoid alcohol during the elimination phase

- ☐ **Espresso or coffee**

  Limit to 1 cup per day during the elimination phase

- ☐ **Tea**

  Black, green, peppermint

FOUR WEEKS TO A HEALTHY GUT + MEAL PLANS + REINTRODUCTION

FOUR-WEEK MEAL PLAN

The following meal plan is intended to be personalized by you. If you prefer to have only one snack each day, then do that. Or eat your snack choice after dinner as a dessert. If you are vegan, then stick to the vegan recipes in this book (there are several).

The recipes vary in serving sizes. If you are making meals for a group, then you may wish to double some of the recipes so that you have leftovers for the next day. If you are cooking for one, then you may wish to freeze items for later.

Side dishes on the meal plan that are not recipes in this book are suggested for you as an accompaniment for some of the meals. Prepare those items as you desire using low-FODMAP seasonings. The goal is for you to succeed *and* enjoy what you are eating.

WEEK ONE

This is the biggest week of the diet, since you will be building the foundation for success in your home. You have gone to the grocery store and organized the ingredients you need, so we are going to put them to work.

There are a few items that you may wish to make either the day before you begin or on the first day. Some of these foods you will enjoy for the entire four weeks.

PEP TALK

If you are fearful of changing your eating: Many people have been living with IBS for so long that they are afraid of eating. Feel free to take it slow and stick to your comfort foods, as long as they are low-FODMAP. Over time, as you feel better, you will find it easier to branch out.

If you are confused: The low-FODMAP diet does not "make sense" to our logic of eating. It is hard to understand why you can't have apples and onions, but you can have oranges and carrots. Give it a chance—it will get easier!

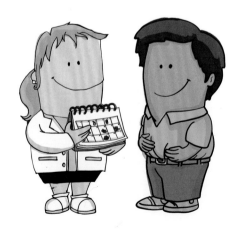

WEEK ONE	Breakfast	Snack 1	Lunch	Snack 2	Dinner
Sunday	Blueberry and Oat Smoothie (page 34)	Scrumptious Pumpkin Pie Energy Bites (page 150)	Classic Chef's Salad (page 58) with The Best Ranch Dressing or Dip (page 168)	½ yellow banana and 1 tablespoon (15 g) peanut butter	No-Bake Chicken Parmesan (page 107) and gluten-free low-FODMAP spaghetti
Monday	French Toast Overnight Oats (page 36)	One-Pot Candied Peanuts (page 149)	Leftover Classic Chef's Salad	Maple and Cinnamon Protein Yogurt (page 155)	Broiled Salmon with Maple Lemon Glaze (page 72) and Perfect Rice Pilaf (page 59)
Tuesday	Tomato, Spinach, and Cheese Handheld Egg Frittatas (page 39) on a low-FODMAP bun	½ cup (75 g) red grapes and 1 stick cheese	2 slices low-FODMAP bread and 5 ounces (140 g) smoked turkey with lettuce, tomato, and mayonnaise and ½ cup (60 g) sliced carrots	2 squares dark chocolate with ½ cup (50 g) low-FODMAP pretzels	One-Pan Maple Mustard Chicken (page 109), baked potato, and steamed broccoli heads
Wednesday	Strawberry, Banana, and Flax Smoothie (page 34)	Scrumptious Pumpkin Pie Energy Bites (page 150)	Leftover One-Pan Maple Mustard Chicken and ½ baked potato	1 orange	Hearty Beef, Quinoa, and Lentil Casserole (page 112) and sautéed spinach
Thursday	Tomato, Spinach, and Cheese Handheld Egg Frittatas (page 39) on a low-FODMAP bun	Lactose-free yogurt and 1 cup (145 g) strawberries	Leftover Hearty Beef, Quinoa, and Lentil Casserole	One-Pot Candied Peanuts (page 149)	Tasty Tuna Salad (page 88) melt with cheese and sliced tomatoes and sliced carrot sticks
Friday	French Toast Overnight Oats (page 36)	4 gluten-free crackers and 1 tablespoon (15 g) almond butter	Leftover Tasty Tuna Salad on low-FODMAP bagel and bag of plain potato chips	½ cup (75 g) grapes	Chicken Breasts with Rosemary and Artichoke Hearts (page 91) and steamed quinoa
Saturday	Fluffy Pancakes with Walnuts and Cinnamon (page 40)	1 cup (120 g) carrot sticks	Leftover Chicken Breasts with Rosemary and Artichoke Hearts and quinoa	Confetti Vanilla Mug Cake (page 143)	Grilled Steak with Soy and Lime (page 96) and Lemon Rosemary New Potatoes (page 70)

WEEK TWO

You have made it through the first week! Congratulations! Keep at it, and your gut will heal with every passing day.

PEP TALK

If you haven't noticed an improvement: Not everyone responds to the low-FODMAP diet in the first week. Be patient. Chances are high (70 to 80 percent) that you will start seeing improvements this week. You can do this!

If it seems really hard: Sticking to any eating program can be cumbersome. Maybe you are accustomed to eating takeout three days a week? Possibly you got a sudden deadline and have to work late? Take a breath and do your best. Your body will thank you.

WEEK TWO	Breakfast	Snack 1	Lunch	Snack 2	Dinner
Sunday	Make-Ahead Breakfast Burritos (page 45)	DIY Trail Mix (page 136)	Flat-Tummy Chicken Corn Chowder (page 56) and low-FODMAP crackers	Creamy Chia Pudding with Coconut (page 139)	Classic Breaded Pork Chops (page 95) and tossed salad with Everyone's Favorite Italian Dressing (page 169)
Monday	French Toast Overnight Oats (page 36)	One-Pot Candied Peanuts (page 149)	Leftover Flat-Tummy Chicken Corn Chowder and low-FODMAP crackers	10 medium sliced strawberries	Broiled Lemon Pepper Cod on Parchment (page 78), steamed quinoa, and sliced cucumbers
Tuesday	Tomato, Spinach, and Cheese Handheld Egg Frittatas (page 39) on a low-FODMAP bun	½ cup (75 g) grapes	2 slices low-FODMAP bread with deli smoked turkey or ham and 1 slice Swiss cheese, lettuce, and tomato	Scrumptious Pumpkin Pie Energy Bites (page 150)	Ten-Minute Spaghetti Sauce (page 116) and low-FODMAP pasta
Wednesday	Peanut Butter and Cinnamon Smoothie (page 35)	1 ounce (28 g) mozzarella cheese and 1 orange	Leftover Ten-Minute Spaghetti Sauce and pasta	Carrot Mug Muffin with Walnuts and Coconut (page 154)	Niçoise Salad (page 67)
Thursday	Make-Ahead Breakfast Burritos (page 45)	DIY Trail Mix (page 136)	Leftover Niçoise Salad	Maple and Cinnamon Protein Yogurt (page 155)	"Better Than Takeout" Chicken Fried Rice (page 113)
Friday	French Toast Overnight Oats (page 36)	One-Pot Candied Peanuts (page 149)	Leftover "Better Than Takeout" Chicken Fried Rice	½ yellow banana and 1 tablespoon (15 g) almond butter	Breaded Miniature Turkey Burgers (page 98) with Copycat Secret Sauce (page 169) and steamed broccoli heads
Saturday	Kale and Cheese Egg Scramble (page 49) and toasted low-FODMAP bread	10 medium sliced strawberries	Hummus Pizza with Greek Salad (page 129)	Intensely Addictive Cornflake Cookies with Chocolate Chips (page 146)	Brown Sugar Foil-Wrapped Salmon (page 89), baked potatoes, and sliced carrots

WEEK THREE

By this point, you are halfway through the meal plan and are getting more adept at the low-FODMAP lifestyle. Don't lose your focus!

PEP TALK

If you are getting bored: You may be craving your favorite lasagna or chicken dinner. Feel free to prepare something you love using a low-FODMAP recipe from a reliable source (like rachelpaulsfood.com or fodmapeveryday.com). Be creative!

If you are losing momentum: It is common to question whether you *truly* need to be on the low-FODMAP diet. Don't test things yet! Wait until the next phase (reintroduction) to check your tolerances.

If you make a mistake: If you have a *slipup*, don't *give* up! Just begin the next day as a fresh start.

WEEK THREE	Breakfast	Snack 1	Lunch	Snack 2	Dinner
Sunday	Pumpkin Pie Breakfast Quinoa (page 48)	Peanut Butter Baked Oatmeal Squares (page 43)	Carrot Soup with Coconut and Curry (page 54) and low-FODMAP crackers	Parmesan and Garlic Gourmet Popcorn (page 142)	The Best Burgers (page 108), sliced tomatoes and lettuce, low-FODMAP buns, and Crispy Baked Garlic French Fries (page 65)
Monday	Protein-Packed Mixed Fruit Smoothie Bowl (page 46)	Scrumptious Pumpkin Pie Energy Bites (page 150)	Leftover Carrot Soup with Coconut and Curry and low-FODMAP crackers	1 ounce (28 g) salted peanuts	Kale and Cabbage Salad with Pepitas (page 58) and grilled chicken breasts marinated with Everyone's Favorite Italian Dressing (page 69)
Tuesday	Tomato, Spinach, and Cheese Handheld Egg Frittatas (page 39) on ½ low-FODMAP bagel	Parmesan and Garlic Gourmet Popcorn (page 142)	Leftover Kale and Cabbage Salad with Pepitas and grilled chicken breast	Intensely Addictive Cornflake Cookies with Chocolate Chips (page 146)	Peanut Pad Thai (page 130)
Wednesday	French Toast Overnight Oats (page 36)	Maple and Cinnamon Protein Yogurt (page 155)	Leftover Peanut Pad Thai	1 orange and 1 stick cheese	Sweet and Savory Shrimp (page 73) and steamed rice
Thursday	Make-Ahead Breakfast Burritos (page 45)	Peanut Butter Baked Oatmeal Squares (page 43)	2 slices low-FODMAP bread with deli smoked turkey and 1 slice Swiss cheese, lettuce, and tomato	10 almonds and ½ cup (75 g) grapes	Mediterranean Chicken with Olives and Tomatoes (page 96) and low-FODMAP penne
Friday	Raspberry and Chia Protein Smoothie (page 35)	One-Pot Candied Peanuts (page 149)	Leftover Mediterranean Chicken with Olives and Tomatoes and low-FODMAP penne	Maple and Cinnamon Protein Yogurt (page 155)	Seared Scallops with Baby Spinach (page 79) and Lemon Rosemary New Potatoes (page 70)
Saturday	Pumpkin Pie Breakfast Quinoa (page 48)	DIY Trail Mix (page 136)	Chickpea Noodle Soup with Spinach (page 55)	Peanut Butter Chocolate Chip Microwave Cookie (page 137)	Crispy Chicken Nuggets (page 104) with Microwave Sweet and Sour Sauce (page 163) and steamed brown rice

WEEK FOUR

You are almost there, and it feels great. But you may be upset or nervous about the future.

PEP TALK

Cancel the "pity party": You may be feeling depressed that you can't have all the foods you love on the low-FODMAP diet. I get that. But think about how lucky you are to have found your IBS solution! Focus on the positives and how great you are feeling.

If you're afraid to stop low-FODMAP eating: You may be concerned about introducing high-FODMAP foods during the next phase of reintroduction. Your gut is happy, and you don't want that to stop. It's fine to wait a little longer. Just realize that the goal is for you to "personalize" a FODMAP-aware way of eating, as a component of your healthiest lifestyle.

WEEK FOUR	Breakfast	Snack 1	Lunch	Snack 2	Dinner
Sunday	Cinnamon Roll Traditional Cooked Oatmeal (page 33)	1 ounce (28 g) salted peanuts	Summertime Salad with Toasted Pecans (page 62) and low-FODMAP bagel with 2 tablespoons (30 g) cream cheese	Chewy Brownie Cookies with Walnuts (page 153)	One-Pan Tilapia with Lemon, Garlic, and Capers (page 73) and low-FODMAP spaghettini or angel hair pasta
Monday	Make-Ahead Breakfast Burritos (page 45)	4 low-FODMAP crackers with 1 tablespoon (15 g) peanut butter	Leftover Summertime Salad with Toasted Pecans, low-FODMAP toast, and "Humm in Your Head" Hummus (page 159)	Protein-Packed Mixed Fruit Smoothie Bowl (page 46)	Quinoa and Lentil Kitchari (page 118)
Tuesday	Pumpkin Spice Smoothie (page 33)	DIY Trail Mix (page 136)	Leftover Quinoa and Lentil Kitchari	Banana Chocolate Chip Oat Bars (page 140)	Roasted Chicken with Spiced Maple Glaze (page 92), steamed rice, and broccoli heads
Wednesday	Blueberry and Oat Smoothie (page 34)	One-Pot Candied peanuts (page 149)	Leftover Roasted Chicken with Spiced Maple Glaze, rice, and broccoli heads	Sliced carrots with The Best Ranch Dressing or Dip (page 168)	Dijon-Crusted Salmon (page 75) and Asian Vegetable Stir-Fry (page 66)
Thursday	Peanut Butter Baked Oatmeal Squares (page 43)	Scrumptious Pumpkin Pie Energy Bites (page 150)	Leftover Asian Vegetable Stir-Fry with 1 cup (185 g) steamed quinoa	½ cup (75 g) red grapes and 1 ounce (28 g) mozzarella cheese	Beef and Spinach Enchiladas (page 100)
Friday	Strawberry, Banana, and Flax Smoothie (page 34)	Banana Chocolate Chip Oat Bars (page 140)	Simply Stuffed Microwave Baked Potato (page 134)	10 almonds and 1 orange	Yummy Pineapple Chicken (page 103) with Perfect Rice Pilaf (page 59)
Saturday	Lemon Blueberry Mug Muffin (page 44)	10 medium sliced strawberries	Leftover Yummy Pineapple Chicken and leftover Perfect Rice Pilaf	DIY Trail Mix (page 136)	Tangy Turkey Sloppy Joes (page 97) with low-FODMAP buns and tossed salad of lettuce, tomatoes, and pumpkin seeds with The Best Ranch Dressing or Dip (page 168)

NEXT STEPS: REINTRODUCTION AND PERSONALIZATION

Reintroduction is the process of figuring out which high-FODMAP foods you are able to tolerate. You will be testing your sensitivity using one food group at a time, in a methodical way, and it can seem scary at first. Each high-FODMAP subgroup should be evaluated individually, as a FODMAP *challenge*, while the rest of your diet remains low in FODMAPs. Since most of us do not know which foods are best to administer for each challenge phase, working with a dietitian is beneficial.

Reintroduction is done slowly and with time between new foods to make sure you are able to detect changes in symptoms. As you reintroduce foods, you may discover that you can tolerate a whole subcategory of FODMAPs (such as lactose), while you can only tolerate some foods in another category. A *failed* challenge is when you experience symptoms typically associated with IBS, such as gas, bloating, diarrhea, or constipation.

Personalization is the final stage of being FODMAP aware. Once you understand which foods your body tolerates, you can personalize an eating plan as part of your permanent lifestyle. Our bodies are always changing, and you may notice an ability to increase your food choices with time.

The best part is, you will be able to tell which foods are triggers for you. *That* is the solution to your IBS, and the key to a forever happy and healthy you.

RECIPE ICONS

 Vegan

 Vegetarian

 Gluten Free

 Dairy Free

 Under 5 Ingredients

 Make Ahead

 One-Pan

 One-Jar

 One-Bowl

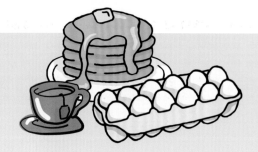

2

EASY BREAKFASTS FOR HOME OR ON THE ROAD

Start your day right with these amazing recipes for smoothies and breakfast favorites. They're easy to prep and eat on the go!

PUMPKIN SPICE SMOOTHIE

This low-FODMAP smoothie is delicious all year-round. Canned pumpkin is a super-convenient way to add nutrition and low-FODMAP flavor to recipes, in servings of ⅓ cup (75 g) per person. FODMAP fact: While bananas are low-FODMAP, pay attention to ripeness and amount. The riper the banana, the higher the FODMAP content. So, for a ripe banana, ⅓ medium banana is a single low-FODMAP serving. However, if the banana is underripe, you can enjoy a whole medium banana.

Place all the ingredients in a blender and blend on high speed until the desired consistency is reached.

NOTE For a low-sugar smoothie, use sucralose or stevia (1 to 2 teaspoons) instead of maple syrup.

TIP If you don't have pumpkin pie spice, you can substitute ½ teaspoon ground cinnamon, ¼ teaspoon ground nutmeg, ⅛ teaspoon ground cloves, and ⅛ teaspoon ground ginger.

⅓ frozen ripe banana

⅓ cup (75 g) canned pure pumpkin puree

1 teaspoon pumpkin pie spice

1 tablespoon (15 ml) pure maple syrup

1 cup (240 ml) low-FODMAP milk (such as 2% lactose-free milk or unsweetened almond milk)

½ cup (120 g) ice cubes (optional)

  Yield: 2 servings   **Prep time:** 2 minutes   **Cook time:** 10 minutes

CINNAMON ROLL TRADITIONAL COOKED OATMEAL

This is the oatmeal that reminds me of breakfast time as a kid. I love "stick to your ribs" stove-top oatmeal, piled high with sugar and cinnamon. You will devour this filling and heart-healthy, low-FODMAP breakfast as it warms you from the inside out.

In a small saucepan, bring the milk to a gentle boil. Stir in the oats, turn the heat to low, and cook until the oats have absorbed the milk, 3 to 5 minutes. Turn off the heat and stir in the cinnamon, vanilla, and brown sugar. Serve immediately.

2 cups (480 ml) low-FODMAP milk (such as 2% lactose-free milk or unsweetened almond milk)

1 cup (80 g) traditional rolled oats

1 teaspoon ground cinnamon

1 teaspoon vanilla extract

3 tablespoons (45 g) brown sugar

VARIATION

+ **Chai Spiced Oatmeal:** Substitute the 1 teaspoon ground cinnamon with ¼ teaspoon ground cinnamon, ⅛ teaspoon ground cardamom, ⅛ teaspoon ground nutmeg, and ⅛ teaspoon ground ginger.

BLUEBERRY AND OAT SMOOTHIE

This creamy smoothie is so easy to make and is packed with nutritional power. Low-FODMAP oats provide healthy fiber, protein, and antioxidants, and keep you feeling full all morning long. Blueberries are a superfood, but pay attention to the serving size for FODMAP levels. If consuming more than ⅓ cup (40 g), there will be higher levels of fructans, which could be harder to digest. This is the reason I love having my kitchen scale handy.

Place all the ingredients in a blender and blend on high speed until the desired consistency is reached.

NOTE For a low-sugar smoothie, use sucralose or stevia (1 to 2 teaspoons) instead of maple syrup.

VARIATION

+ For higher protein content, add 1 scoop of your favorite low-FODMAP protein powder.

1½ cups (360 ml) low-FODMAP milk (such as 2% lactose-free milk or unsweetened almond milk)

⅓ cup (40 g) blueberries (fresh or frozen)

½ cup (40 g) traditional rolled oats

1½ tablespoons (23 ml) maple syrup

½ teaspoon vanilla extract

STRAWBERRY, BANANA, AND FLAX SMOOTHIE

Strawberries are an incredible fruit for low-FODMAP eating. You can enjoy a whopping 10 medium strawberries (150 g) per serving. I love the color and flavor of a strawberry smoothie. Using flaxseed meal gives this smoothie thickness, fiber, and omega-3 nutrition.

Place all the ingredients in a blender and blend on high speed until the desired consistency is reached.

NOTE For a low-sugar smoothie, use sucralose or stevia (1 to 2 teaspoons) instead of maple syrup.

VARIATION

+ For a thicker smoothie, opt for ½ cup (120 g) coconut yogurt (vegan) or lactose-free yogurt (non-vegan) to replace ½ cup (120 ml) of the low-FODMAP milk.

1½ cups (360 ml) low-FODMAP milk (such as 2% lactose-free milk or unsweetened almond milk)

1 cup (150 g) strawberries

⅓ medium frozen ripe banana

1 tablespoon (7 g) flaxseed meal

1½ tablespoons (23 ml) maple syrup

RASPBERRY AND CHIA PROTEIN SMOOTHIE

I love that raspberries are safe for the low-FODMAP diet. They are packed with fiber and can be consumed at servings of ½ cup (60 g), or about 30 berries. Adding chia seeds provides even more fiber, protein, and omega-3 fats. This smoothie will keep you feeling full for hours!

Place all the ingredients in a blender and blend on high speed until the desired consistency is reached.

NOTE For a low-sugar smoothie, use sucralose or stevia (1 to 2 teaspoons) instead of maple syrup.

TIP I prefer brown rice protein powder due to its low-FODMAP ingredients. Be careful to avoid protein powders with inulin, fruit extracts, or sorbitol.

1½ cups (360 ml) low-FODMAP milk (such as 2% lactose-free milk or unsweetened almond milk)

½ cup (60 g) raspberries

1 tablespoon (8 g) chia seeds

1 tablespoon (8 g) low-FODMAP protein powder

1½ tablespoons (23 ml) maple syrup

   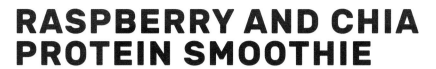 **Yield:** 15 ounces (420 ml), 1 to 2 servings   **Prep time:** 5 minutes

PEANUT BUTTER AND CINNAMON SMOOTHIE

This peanut butter smoothie is creamy and absolutely delicious. Peanut butter is a healthy and inexpensive low-FODMAP food option, which you can enjoy in servings of 2 tablespoons (30 g). FODMAP fact: While almond butter is also low-FODMAP, you must limit servings to 1 tablespoon (15 g) due to a higher FODMAP level in almonds.

Place all the ingredients in a blender and blend on high speed until the desired consistency is reached.

NOTE In case of peanut allergies, substitute 2 tablespoons (30 g) sunflower seed butter for the peanut butter.

TIP For a low-sugar smoothie, use sucralose or stevia (1 to 2 teaspoons) instead of maple syrup.

VARIATION

✦ If you like peanut butter and banana, add ⅓ frozen banana to the smoothie.

1½ cups (360 ml) low-FODMAP milk (such as 2% lactose-free milk or unsweetened almond milk)

½ cup (120 g) plain low-FODMAP yogurt (such as lactose-free yogurt or coconut yogurt)

2 tablespoons (30 g) all-natural smooth peanut butter (salted or unsalted)

1½ tablespoons (23 ml) maple syrup

1 teaspoon ground cinnamon

EASY BREAKFASTS FOR HOME OR ON THE ROAD

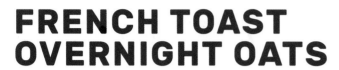
FRENCH TOAST OVERNIGHT OATS

Overnight oats are an amazing low-FODMAP breakfast for on-the-go mornings. Individual mason jars make it simple to prep, clean up, and eat on the run. Traditional rolled oats are low-FODMAP in ½-cup (52 g) servings, which makes a lot of oatmeal when it has the time to expand, creating a filling, high-fiber, and healthy meal choice that tastes sensational.

½ cup (120 ml) low-FODMAP milk (such as 2% lactose-free milk or unsweetened almond milk)

½ cup (52 g) traditional (old-fashioned) rolled oats

1 tablespoon (15 ml) pure maple syrup

1½ teaspoons chia seeds

½ teaspoon ground cinnamon

1 tablespoon (8 g) low-FODMAP protein powder

Place all the ingredients in a mason jar or other covered bowl and stir well to combine. Leave overnight in the refrigerator. Can be served cold or warmed in the microwave.

NOTE Switch out the maple syrup for sucralose or stevia (2 to 3 teaspoons) if you are cutting calories.

TIP Double or triple this recipe to have breakfast for multiple mornings. These overnight oats will keep in the refrigerator for 5 days.

VARIATION

+ Top with chopped almonds, peanuts, sliced banana, or more maple syrup.

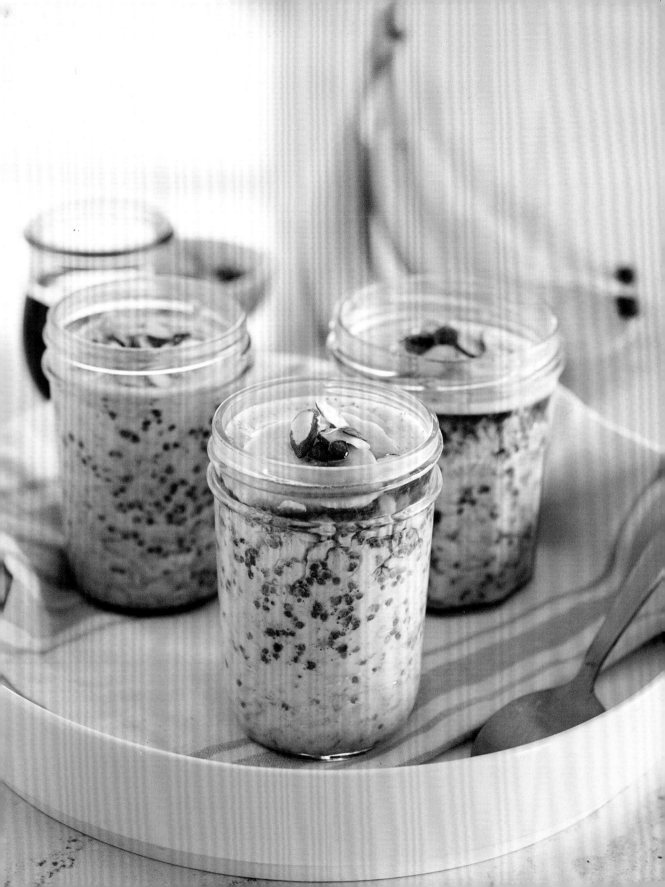

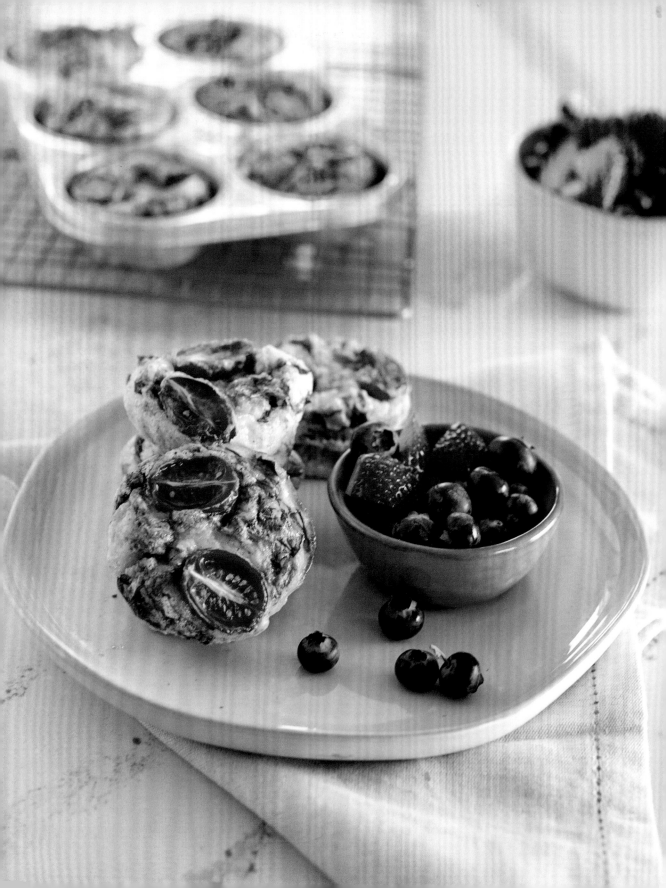

TOMATO, SPINACH, AND CHEESE HANDHELD EGG FRITTATAS

These mini frittatas are the perfect handheld sandwich; they are delicious, filling, and so good for you. Spinach is a superfood—it provides iron, vitamins, and minerals—while the cheese and eggs are wonderful protein sources. FODMAP facts: Cheese is naturally low in lactose, which makes it a versatile low-FODMAP food choice. You can also enjoy up to 1½ cups (75 g) baby spinach as a low-FODMAP serving.

Preheat the oven to 350°F (180°C or gas mark 4) and place a rack in the center of the oven. Coat a 12-cup muffin tin with vegetable shortening or spray with nonstick cooking spray.

In a large bowl, whisk the eggs until light and frothy. Add the salt, pepper, and paprika. Divide the egg mixture among the muffin cups, filling them about halfway to two-thirds full, depending on the size of your muffin tin. Divide the three toppings evenly among the muffin cups: 1 tomato, 1 tablespoon (3 g) spinach, and 2 tablespoons (16 g) cheese for each. Bake for 15 to 20 minutes, until the center is set and no longer jiggles.

Remove from the oven and let cool for about 3 minutes in the tin. Loosen around the edges and scoop out each frittata onto a serving plate. Add more salt and pepper to taste. Serve in a gluten-free low-FODMAP bun or alongside low-FODMAP fruit.

Vegetable shortening or nonstick cooking spray

12 large eggs

¼ teaspoon salt, plus more to taste

¼ teaspoon freshly ground pepper, plus more to taste

⅛ teaspoon paprika

12 cherry tomatoes, halved or quartered

¾ cup (38 g) fresh spinach, coarsely chopped

1½ cups (180 g) shredded mozzarella or sharp Cheddar cheese

TIP *To make ahead:* **Once cooled, these can be stored in the refrigerator for 3 days, or frozen for longer. If freezing, wrap well in plastic wrap surrounded by aluminum foil. When ready to eat, remove from the foil and plastic and wrap in a slightly dampened paper towel. Microwave for 45 to 90 seconds, checking and turning every 30 seconds.**

FLUFFY PANCAKES WITH WALNUTS AND CINNAMON

This recipe is a family favorite, modified from my mother's recipe. Pancakes are the best weekend meal and are easily made low-FODMAP. Gluten-free pancake/biscuit mix is a pantry staple for me, because it has xanthan gum and baking powder added already. Toasting the walnuts makes them taste so much better. These pancakes are light and fluffy, with crispy edges and a delicious flavor. So easy and so good.

1 egg

¾ cup plus 2 tablespoons (210 ml) low-FODMAP milk (such as 2% lactose-free milk or unsweetened almond milk)

1 cup (120 g) gluten-free low-FODMAP pancake/biscuit mix, homemade (page 44) or store-bought

½ teaspoon vanilla extract

1 teaspoon ground cinnamon

1 cup (95 g) chopped walnuts, toasted (see Tip)

Canola oil, for frying

Crack the egg into a large mixing bowl, and whisk well. Add about ¼ cup (60 ml) of the milk and whisk again until blended. Begin incorporating the gluten-free pancake mix a little at a time, alternating with the milk, until well incorporated (for thinner pancakes, add more milk, 1 tablespoon [15 ml] at a time, until your desired consistency is reached). Add the vanilla and cinnamon and stir together. Fold in the toasted walnut pieces.

Place a large skillet over medium heat and add about 1 teaspoon of canola oil. When the oil is hot, ladle the batter into the skillet, about ¼ cup (60 ml) per pancake. Cook until the edges are crispy, then flip gently with a spatula. When the second side is cooked, transfer to a plate to keep warm until all the pancakes are finished. Repeat until the batter is gone, adding more oil as needed. Serve immediately or store in the refrigerator, covered, for 2 days.

NOTE Serve these pancakes with maple syrup, butter, and your favorite low-FODMAP fruit on the side.

TIP *To toast nuts:* Preheat the oven to 350°F (180°C or gas mark 4). Spread the nuts in a single layer on a baking sheet and bake for 10 to 15 minutes, until browned. I do this with all my nuts and seeds, then tuck them in my freezer until a recipe calls for them.

VARIATION

✤ Swap the walnuts for blueberries, banana, or chocolate chips, or just enjoy plain.

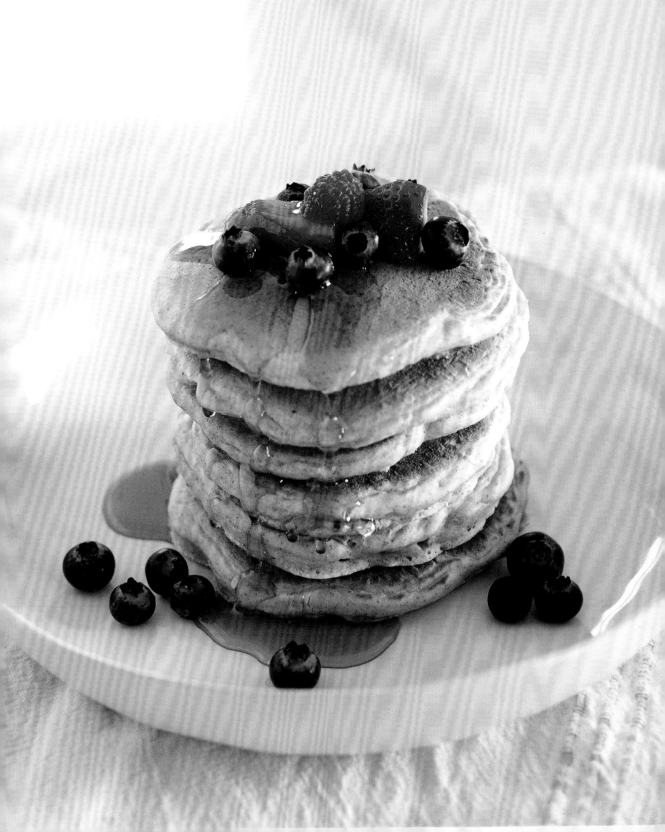

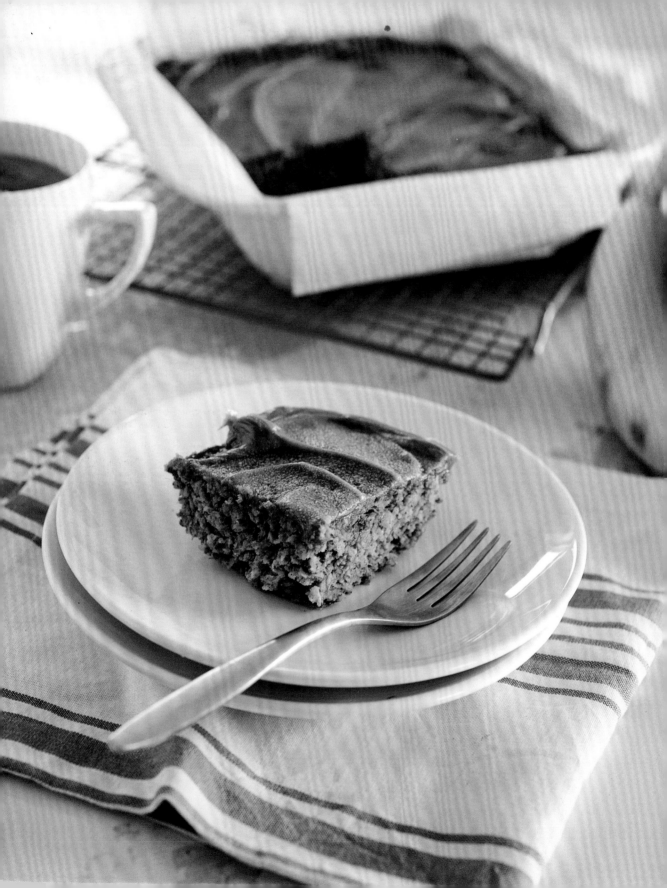

PEANUT BUTTER BAKED OATMEAL SQUARES

These baked oatmeal squares are amazing anytime. They provide the protein of peanuts, the fiber of oats, and the minerals of banana. FODMAP fact: Quick oats are low-FODMAP in ¼-cup (23 g) servings, which is different from traditional rolled oats, where one serving is ½ cup (52 g).

Preheat the oven to 350°F (180°C or gas mark 4) and place a rack in the center of the oven. Grease an 8 x 8-inch (20 x 20 cm) square baking pan and line with parchment paper, leaving a 2-inch (5 cm) overhang on the sides. Grease the parchment paper as well.

In a small bowl, combine the oats, baking powder, salt, and cinnamon. Set aside.

In a large bowl, combine the mashed banana and ¼ cup (60 g) of the peanut butter. Add the vanilla, ½ cup (120 ml) of the maple syrup, and the beaten egg. Mix again. Add the low-FODMAP milk and stir until the batter is smooth. Add the dry oat mixture to the wet ingredients and mix thoroughly. Pour the mixture into the prepared pan and smooth the surface with a spatula. Bake for 25 minutes. When done, remove from the oven and let cool for 2 to 3 minutes.

Meanwhile, stir the remaining 1 tablespoon (15 ml) maple syrup into the remaining ¼ cup (60 g) peanut butter until smooth and spread over the warm oatmeal. Cut into 12 rectangles and enjoy warm, or refrigerate until serving (tastes great hot or cold). These can also be frozen wrapped individually in squares.

TIP Vegans, try this egg substitute: Dissolve 1 tablespoon (7 g) flaxseed meal in 3 tablespoons (45 ml) warm water and let stand for 20 minutes until it becomes gelatinous. Then use in place of the egg.

Vegetable shortening, for greasing

1½ cups (138 g) quick oats (not traditional rolled oats)

1 teaspoon baking powder

½ teaspoon salt

1 teaspoon ground cinnamon

2 ripe bananas, mashed

½ cup (120 g) all-natural smooth peanut butter, divided

1 teaspoon vanilla extract

½ cup plus 1 tablespoon (135 ml) pure maple syrup, divided

1 egg, lightly beaten

¾ cup (180 ml) low-FODMAP milk (such as 2% lactose-free milk or unsweetened almond milk)

EASY BREAKFASTS FOR HOME OR ON THE ROAD

VARIATION

+ Sprinkle ¼ cup (40 g) semisweet chocolate chips over the top while still warm.

LEMON BLUEBERRY MUG MUFFIN

I love the combination of lemon and blueberries. This mug muffin has the perfect amount of fresh lemon to give it that refreshing tartness. Just right for your morning sunshine wake-up call! A fresh baked muffin in the morning puts a smile on my face for the whole day.

1 egg (you will use 2 tablespoons [30 ml] of whisked egg for this recipe)

3 tablespoons (36 g) sugar, plus more for sprinkling (optional)

3 tablespoons (45 ml) freshly squeezed lemon juice (about ¾ medium lemon)

5 tablespoons (40 g) gluten-free low-FODMAP pancake/biscuit mix, homemade (see Tip) or store-bought

2 tablespoons and 1 teaspoon (35 ml) canola oil

¼ teaspoon vanilla extract

3 tablespoons (30 g) fresh blueberries

Ground cinnamon, for sprinkling (optional)

Crack the egg into a cup and whisk well. Measure out 2 tablespoons (30 ml) of whisked egg into a 12-ounce (360 g) or larger microwave-safe mug and discard or set aside the unused egg for another recipe. Add the sugar and whisk to combine well. Slowly add the lemon juice to the egg mixture. Add the pancake mix, canola oil, and vanilla and mix until blended. Fold in the blueberries, ensuring they are below the surface of the batter so that they don't spatter during cooking. Sprinkle with cinnamon and sugar, if desired. Microwave for 1 minute 15 seconds to 1 minute 30 seconds (should not bubble over). Enjoy immediately.

NOTE If you have only frozen blueberries, rinse them under water to defrost them and minimize bleeding of the juice into the muffin.

TIPS *Bonus recipe!* I like gluten-free Bisquick mix, but if you don't have it, you can make your own. For 1 cup (120 g) copycat gluten-free pancake mix, combine 1 cup (120 g) gluten-free low-FODMAP flour, 1 teaspoon xanthan gum, ½ teaspoon baking soda, 1 teaspoon baking powder, and 1 teaspoon sugar.

To make ahead: Combine all the dry ingredients in a mug the night before, squeeze your lemon juice, and weigh the blueberries. Then you can mix everything together for a delicious fresh-tasting mug muffin, even if you are running late!

VARIATION

+ If you prefer a less lemony muffin, substitute 1 to 2 tablespoons (15 to 30 ml) low-FODMAP milk for the equivalent amount of lemon juice.

MAKE-AHEAD BREAKFAST BURRITOS

Breakfast burritos are my favorite way to enjoy a hot and filling breakfast with minimal preparation. These burritos can be made ahead and frozen in batches. FODMAP fact: Corn tortillas are naturally low-FODMAP, provided they don't contain added wheat or seasonings.

In a large skillet, heat 1 tablespoon (15 ml) of the oil over medium-high heat. Add the shredded potatoes in an even layer and press down with a spatula. Cook for 5 to 7 minutes, then flip and cook the other side. Add another 1 tablespoon (15 ml) oil and cook until browned and crispy throughout. Transfer to a covered bowl to keep warm. Wipe out the skillet.

In a large bowl, whisk the eggs with the paprika. Add the remaining 1 tablespoon (15 ml) oil to the skillet and sauté the red pepper for 2 minutes. Pour the whisked eggs over the peppers and scramble for about 2 minutes, until cooked through. Season liberally with salt and pepper.

To assemble the burritos, lay the tortillas on a platter and top with the potatoes, then the egg mixture, then the cheese. Roll up and serve with salsa, if desired, or freeze (see Tip).

NOTE Not all corn tortillas are alike. Some are fragile and work better for a cooked quesadilla (page 123). Warming the tortilla first can improve the ease of wrapping and reduce tears. Experiment with the brands that you can find and be patient!

TIP *To make-ahead:* After cooling the components, wrap each burrito in aluminum foil. Transfer rolled burritos to a large resealable freezer plastic bag. Remove as much air as possible and freeze for up to 1 month. To reheat, remove a burrito from the foil and wrap in a lightly dampened paper towel. Place on a microwavable plate and microwave on high for 1½ to 2½ minutes, turning once, until heated through.

3 tablespoons (45 ml) canola oil, divided

4 cups (480 g) shredded potatoes

8 eggs

½ teaspoon paprika

½ red bell pepper, chopped

Salt and pepper to taste

Eight 6-inch (15 cm) soft corn tortillas or gluten-free low-FODMAP flour tortillas

2 cups (240 g) shredded Cheddar cheese

Restaurant-Style Salsa (page 161), for serving (optional)

VARIATION

+ For a meat lover's option, fry 8 to 16 strips of bacon or 1 pound (455 g) of ground sausage (before making the eggs). Divide the meat among the burritos.

EASY BREAKFASTS FOR HOME OR ON THE ROAD

PROTEIN-PACKED MIXED FRUIT SMOOTHIE BOWL

Bored of your usual smoothie and want to try something you eat with a spoon? A smoothie bowl is the perfect solution! This smoothie bowl is packed with protein from the yogurt, nut butter, protein powder, and oats. It is so creamy and delicious, and my kids adore it. FODMAP fact: Although raspberries, blueberries, and strawberries are wonderful low-FODMAP berry choices, stay away from blackberries, as they are not low-FODMAP.

½ cup (120 g) plain low-FODMAP yogurt (such as lactose-free yogurt or coconut yogurt)

1½ tablespoons (23 ml) maple syrup

½ cup (50 g) frozen or fresh mixed berries (5 blueberries, 7 raspberries, and 3 strawberries)

⅓ frozen or fresh banana

1 tablespoon (15 g) almond butter

1 tablespoon (8 g) gluten-free low-FODMAP protein powder

2 tablespoons (10 g) traditional rolled oats

1 teaspoon chia seeds

Combine the yogurt, maple syrup, berries, banana, almond butter, and protein powder in a blender and blend on high speed for about 1 minute. Serve in a bowl topped with the rolled oats and chia seeds.

TIP Freeze your blueberries, raspberries, and strawberries in the summertime in resealable bags to always have them ready for smoothies.

VARIATION

+ Instead of the mixed berries, use 1 cup (140 g) chopped fresh pineapple and sprinkle with toasted coconut in place of the oats. Instant tropical smoothie bowl!

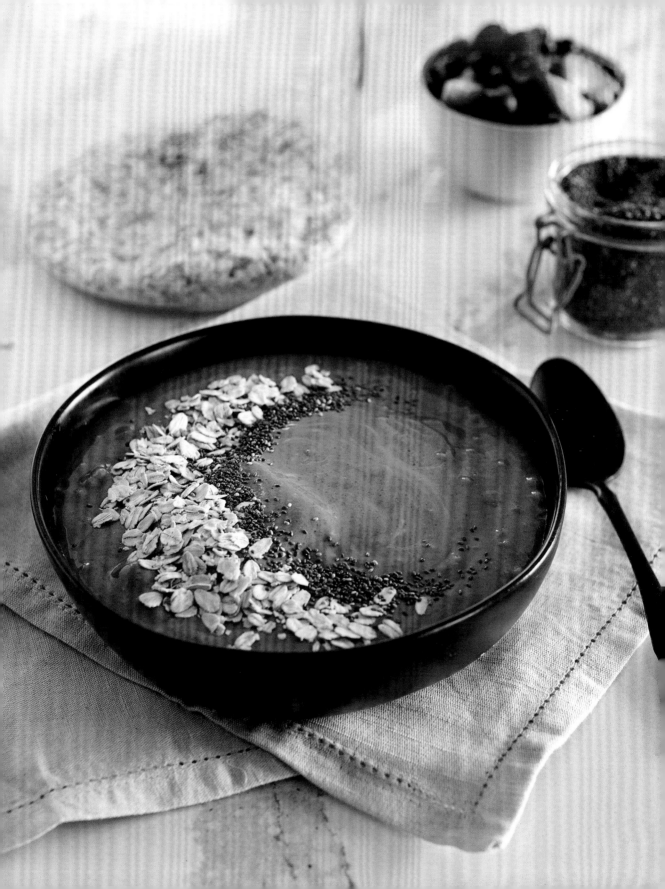

PUMPKIN PIE BREAKFAST QUINOA

Quinoa is an ancient grain and a complete protein source, which means it contains all twenty amino acids. Not only is it healthy and filling, but it is also delicious! I love using quinoa instead of oats or rice for a slightly different texture in my cooking. Cooked quinoa is low-FODMAP in servings of 1 cup (155 g) and is a great choice for vegans.

1 cup (173 g) white quinoa, rinsed

1 cup (240 ml) water

1 cup (240 ml) low-FODMAP milk (such as 2% lactose-free milk or unsweetened almond milk)

1 cup (240 g) canned pumpkin puree

3 tablespoons (45 ml) maple syrup

1 teaspoon pumpkin pie spice

1 teaspoon vanilla extract

In a large saucepan, bring the quinoa, water, and milk to a boil over medium-high heat. Reduce the heat to low, then cover and simmer until the quinoa softens, about 10 minutes. Remove from the heat and stir in the pumpkin puree, syrup, pumpkin pie spice, and vanilla. Serve immediately or refrigerate in mason jars for healthy, on-the-go eating.

NOTE For a creamier quinoa, use canned coconut milk as the milk choice.

TIPS

+ If you don't have pumpkin pie spice, see page 33 for a homemade version.

+ You can substitute brown sugar for the maple syrup.

VARIATION

+ This quinoa is perfect topped with 1 tablespoon (7 g) of toasted pecans.

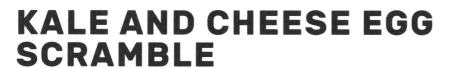
KALE AND CHEESE EGG SCRAMBLE

This is a simple but satisfying breakfast, brunch, or anytime meal. My husband requested this scramble for dinner the other day! Kale is an amazing source of nutrients: 1 cup (67 g) contains 3 grams of protein, 2.6 grams of fiber, and only 33 calories—what a superfood! Only trace FODMAPs are found in kale, so you can enjoy plenty of this healthy treat. I love using kale in salads, stir-fries, and egg scrambles. FODMAP fact: Cheese is naturally low in lactose, so you can enjoy about ⅓ cup (40 g) for one low-FODMAP serving of most cheeses.

Heat the olive oil in a large frying pan over medium-high heat. Add the kale to the pan and cook for a few minutes, until the kale is just wilted. Lower the heat to medium and add the beaten eggs to the pan. Stir until the eggs begin to set. Sprinkle the shredded mozzarella cheese and Italian seasoning over the eggs. Remove from the heat and continue to stir a few times until the cheese is melted and the eggs are cooked. Sprinkle with salt and pepper to taste. Serve immediately.

NOTE This scramble goes perfectly with gluten-free low-FODMAP toast or toasted white sourdough bread (read all about sourdough bread and FODMAPs on page 126) and sliced tomatoes.

TIP *Bonus recipe!* If you don't have low-FODMAP Italian seasoning, you can make your own version. To make 1½ teaspoons of Italian seasoning, use ½ teaspoon dried basil, ½ teaspoon dried oregano, ¼ teaspoon dried rosemary, and ¼ teaspoon dried thyme.

1 tablespoon (15 ml) olive oil

1 cup (67 g) fresh kale, stemmed and chopped

4 eggs, beaten

½ cup (60 g) grated mozzarella cheese

½ teaspoon Italian seasoning, homemade (see Tip) or store-bought

Salt and freshly ground pepper to taste

EASY BREAKFASTS FOR HOME OR ON THE ROAD

VARIATION

+ Switch out the kale for spinach and the mozzarella for Cheddar, and you have a spinach and Cheddar scramble instead!

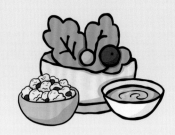

3

SIMPLE STARTERS AND SIDES

These low-FODMAP recipes are perfect for lunch, dinner, and anytime in between.

CAPRESE SALAD WITH BALSAMIC REDUCTION

Who doesn't love a caprese salad? It looks fancy, tastes like heaven, and takes only a few minutes to prepare. You can skip the balsamic reduction to make it even easier. FODMAP facts: Cheese is naturally low in lactose because it contains few carbohydrates. But, beware of the high fat content, because that could also be an IBS trigger. Balsamic vinegar is low-FODMAP in servings of 1 tablespoon (15 ml).

To make the balsamic reduction, if desired: In a large saucepan, bring the balsamic vinegar to a gentle simmer over medium to medium-low heat, stirring occasionally, until it is reduced in volume by half, about 15 minutes. Adjust the heat as necessary to avoid scorching. Remove from the heat and let cool while preparing the other salad ingredients. You will use 2 to 3 tablespoons (30 to 45 ml) for this recipe; store the remaining reduction in a tightly sealed container in the refrigerator.

To make the salad: Arrange the tomatoes and mozzarella in an alternating fashion on a platter, with basil in between each. Drizzle with the olive oil and 2 to 3 tablespoons (30 to 45 ml) of the balsamic reduction and season with salt and pepper.

NOTES

+ High-quality fresh mozzarella makes a real difference in this recipe, so discuss with your favorite grocer to select the best flavor.

+ Vine-ripened and hothouse tomatoes should have a deep consistent red color when ripe and not feel mushy to the touch. They should also have an earthy smell near the stem. For best results, store tomatoes at room temperature in a brown paper bag away from sunlight.

FOR THE BALSAMIC REDUCTION (OPTIONAL)

1 cup (240 ml) balsamic vinegar

FOR THE SALAD

4 vine-ripened tomatoes (about 2 pounds [900 g]), cut into ¼-inch (6 mm)-thick slices

1 pound (454 g) fresh mozzarella, cut into ¼-inch (6 mm)-thick slices

1 bunch (20 leaves) fresh basil

2 tablespoons (30 ml) extra virgin olive oil

Sea salt and freshly ground pepper to taste

VARIATION

+ If you like a sweeter balsamic reduction, add 1 to 2 tablespoons (12 to 24 g) of sugar before heating.

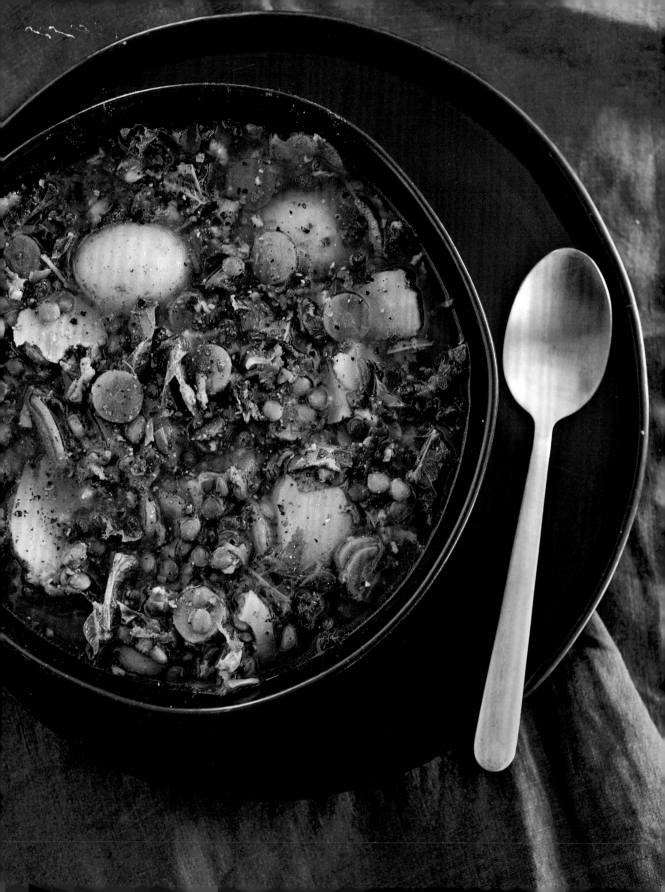

SLOW COOKER BACON, POTATO, AND LENTIL SOUP

This soup is an instant classic. Hearty and flavorful, it reminds me of a split pea soup with bacon (but because peas are not low-FODMAP, I used lentils instead). The ingredients are easy to throw together, and your slow cooker does the rest. Set it up to cook overnight or while you run errands during the day. FODMAP fact: Regular cooked lentils are low-FODMAP in 2-tablespoon (23 g) servings. However, you can enjoy more of the canned variety because the FODMAPs leach into the liquid that is drained off. Therefore, ¼ cup (46 g) of canned lentils is one low-FODMAP serving.

Place the bacon on a microwave-safe plate, cover with paper towels, and microwave until crisp, about 4 minutes, then crumble into pieces.

Place the cooked bacon, potatoes, carrots, lentils, parsnips, stock, and oil in a 5- or 6-quart (4.5 or 5.4 L) slow cooker and cook on low until the potatoes are tender, 6 to 8 hours. Taste the broth and season liberally with salt and pepper. Stir in the kale and cook for about 2 minutes more. Stir in the lemon juice and season with additional salt and pepper as needed.

NOTE For a thicker broth, once the potatoes are cooked, mash about half of the potatoes with a fork inside the slow cooker, then simmer for another 5 minutes before serving.

8 slices thick-cut bacon (uncooked)

2 pounds (910 g) baby Yukon gold potatoes, halved

1 cup (120 g) sliced carrots (¼-inch [6 mm] coins)

½ cup (92 g) dried lentils (will yield 1¼ cups [230 g] cooked lentils)

1 cup (120 g) sliced parsnips (¼-inch [6 mm] coins)

8 cups (1920 ml) low-FODMAP chicken stock, homemade (page 167) or store-bought (page 21)

2 tablespoons (30 ml) garlic-infused olive oil (page 25)

Salt and pepper to taste

3 cups (210 g) chopped kale, stemmed

2 tablespoons (30 ml) freshly squeezed lemon juice (about ½ medium lemon)

VARIATION

+ For vegetarians/vegans, use low-FODMAP vegan stock and omit the bacon.

SIMPLE STARTERS AND SIDES

CARROT SOUP WITH COCONUT AND CURRY

This is a creamy and delicious soup that I crave all year long. Infused olive oils are my favorite way to add flavors of garlic and onion, without FODMAPs. See page 21 for the reason!

3 tablespoons (45 ml) infused olive oil (onion- or garlic-infused, or a combination of both, see page 25)

12 ounces (340 g) carrots, peeled and cut into ½-inch (1.3 cm) coins

1 teaspoon peeled, grated fresh ginger

2 to 3 cups (480 to 720 ml) low-FODMAP vegan or chicken stock, homemade (page 167) or store-bought (page 21)

½ cup (120 ml) low-FODMAP milk (such as 2% lactose-free milk or unsweetened almond milk)

½ cup (120 ml) canned coconut cream (see Note)

1 teaspoon yellow curry powder

⅛ teaspoon cayenne pepper

½ teaspoon salt

½ teaspoon freshly ground pepper

Chopped fresh cilantro, for garnish (optional)

Heat the oil in a heavy saucepan or Dutch oven over medium heat. Add the carrots and ginger, stir, and cook until softened, about 10 minutes. Add 2 cups (480 ml) of the stock; there should be enough to cover the carrots. Bring the mixture to a boil over high heat. Reduce the heat to medium and continue cooking until the carrots are cooked through, 10 to 15 minutes. Add the milk, canned coconut cream, curry powder, cayenne, salt, and pepper and stir to combine.

If you have an immersion blender, puree the soup in the pot; if not, wait until the soup cools slightly, and then puree in a food processor or blender. Add as much of the remaining 1 cup (240 ml) stock to bring the soup to the consistency you want, and season with more salt and pepper to taste. Serve immediately, garnished with fresh cilantro, if desired.

NOTES

+ Select yellow curry powder without onion or garlic. If not available, substitute ½ teaspoon ground cumin, ½ teaspoon ground turmeric, and ½ teaspoon ground coriander.

+ Coconut cream is sold canned, or you can substitute a can of full-fat coconut milk. Chill the coconut milk to separate the cream, and scoop it out with a spoon.

+ This soup freezes well. Freeze individual portions in portable microwave-safe containers and have meals ready for the week ahead.

CHICKPEA NOODLE SOUP WITH SPINACH

A variation on traditional chicken noodle, this soup has delicious flavor and texture from the chickpeas. FODMAP fact: Canned chickpeas contain fewer FODMAPs than regular dried chickpeas, because the FODMAPs leach into the liquid that you drain away. You can enjoy ¼-cup (42 g) serving of canned chickpeas, but avoid substituting dried chickpeas in this recipe.

Combine the infused oil, carrots, and thyme in a large soup pot and sauté over medium-high heat until the carrots soften, 5 to 7 minutes. Add 1 tablespoon (15 ml) of the stock if needed to prevent burning. Stir in the flour and continue to cook over medium heat, stirring constantly, for another 2 minutes. Add the remaining stock, cover the pot, and bring to a boil. Once boiling, add the spaghetti, breaking the strands in half as you do so. Decrease the heat to a simmer and cook, partially covered, for another 5 to 10 minutes, until the pasta is al dente (do not overcook, as gluten-free pastas get mushy). Add the chickpeas and continue to simmer for another 3 minutes. Add the spinach and cook for 1 more minute, just until the spinach is wilted. Turn off the heat and add the lemon juice, salt, and pepper. Serve immediately.

1 tablespoon (15 ml) garlic-infused olive oil (page 25)

3 medium carrots, diced

¾ teaspoon dried thyme

8 cups (1920 ml) low-FODMAP vegan stock, divided

1 tablespoon (8 g) all-purpose gluten-free low-FODMAP flour

8 ounces (224 g) uncooked gluten-free low-FODMAP spaghetti

1½ cups (252 g) canned chickpeas, drained and rinsed

2 cups (60 g) baby spinach

1 tablespoon (15 ml) freshly squeezed lemon juice (about ½ small lemon)

Salt and pepper to taste

VARIATIONS

+ Try this with gluten-free low-FODMAP elbow macaroni or penne for a different texture and experience.

+ For non-vegans, grate some Parmesan cheese over the top for a little extra flavor.

SIMPLE STARTERS AND SIDES

55

FLAT-TUMMY CHICKEN CORN CHOWDER

This is a great soup for all seasons. Light but filling, it's a chowder that won't weigh you down. I love using carrots and parsnips in my low-FODMAP cooking because they are so delicious and good for you. FODMAP facts: Carrots and parsnips do not contain FODMAPs, so you can enjoy as much as you like. Sweet corn, however, can be high in FODMAPs when it comes from a can. Stick with fresh corn off a cob in individual servings of ⅓ cup (40 g) at a time.

2 tablespoons (30 ml) garlic-infused olive oil (page 25)

2 large carrots, peeled and chopped into small cubes

1 parsnip, peeled and chopped into thin slices

6 cups (1440 ml) low-FODMAP chicken stock, homemade (page 167) or store-bought (page 21)

12 ounces (340 g) cooked, diced chicken breast (ensure no high-FODMAP seasonings if bought precooked)

¾ cup (90 g) fresh or fresh frozen corn (not canned)

Salt and pepper to taste

Heat the oil in a large saucepan over medium-high heat. Add the carrots and parsnip and cook, stirring occasionally, until heated through, about 5 minutes. Add the chicken stock, bring to a simmer, and cook for 10 minutes. Add the chicken and corn, then season with salt and pepper to taste. Cook until the chicken is warmed through, then serve.

NOTE This soup refrigerates well and can be packed into containers for a light and filling weekday lunch.

TIP When making corn on the cob, throw a few extras in the pot and then slice off the kernels and freeze for later use in recipes.

VARIATIONS

+ Try this soup with cooked shrimp, chunked cod, or another white fish instead of chicken.

+ For a creamier soup, replace ½ cup (120 ml) of stock with ½ cup (120 ml) of canned coconut milk.

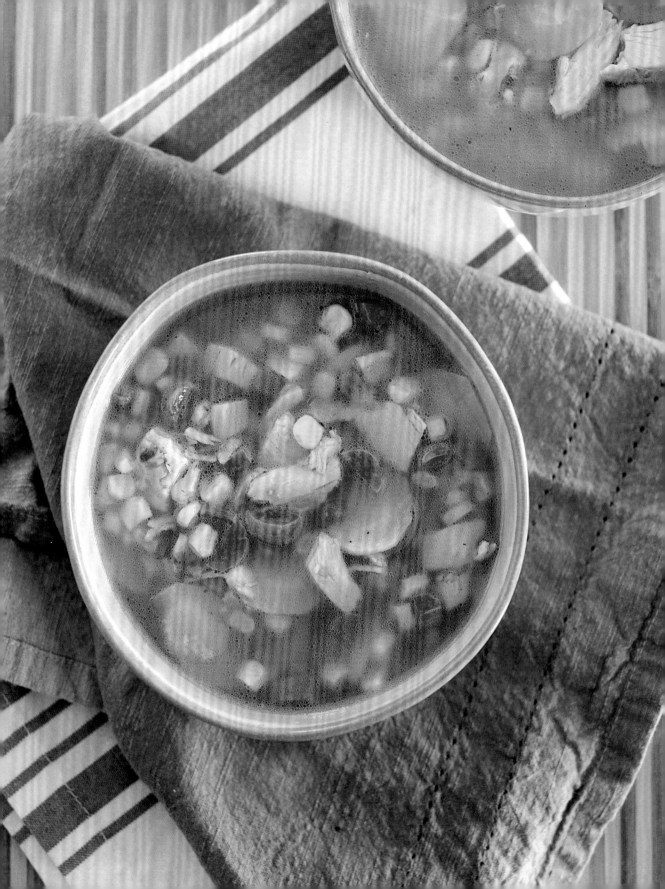

KALE AND CABBAGE SALAD WITH PEPITAS

Did you know you can still enjoy cabbage? FODMAP fact: Red and green cabbage are low-FODMAP in servings of ¾ cup (75 g) at a time. A great way to add color and texture to this delicious salad.

1 bunch kale

1 cup (100 g) sliced red cabbage

1 cup (100 g) sliced green cabbage

1 cup (240 g) hearts of palm (can or jar), chopped

1 medium cucumber, chopped

6 to 8 tablespoons (90 to 120 ml) Sensational Soy Maple Dressing (page 159)

½ cup (55 g) toasted pumpkin seeds (pepitas)

Wash and dry the kale and remove the tough stalks and center veins. Massage the kale with your fingers for about 5 minutes to soften the leaves. Chop the kale. Place the kale, cabbages, hearts of palm, and cucumber in a large bowl, toss with the dressing, and garnish with the pepitas before serving.

NOTE Massaging the kale for 5 minutes will soften the leaves, improve the color, and make the texture and taste even better.

VARIATION

+ Use Sesame Ginger Dressing or Marinade (page 164) instead.

CLASSIC CHEF'S SALAD

Chef's salads are one of my favorite choices, especially in restaurants (ask for oil and vinegar dressing). This salad is packed with protein and super easy to whip up. FODMAP fact: Butter lettuce is a FODMAP-free food, so enjoy as much as you wish.

10 ounces (280 g) cherry tomatoes, halved

6 cups (180 g) butter lettuce, torn or chopped

6 ounces (168 g) cooked and cubed ham (deli style is fine)

8 ounces (224 g) cooked and cubed chicken breast or turkey (deli style is fine)

4 ounces (112 g) cubed or shredded Cheddar cheese

5 hard-boiled eggs, cut in half

½ cup (120 ml) The Best Ranch Dressing or Dip (page 168)

Arrange the tomatoes, lettuce, ham, chicken, cheese, and eggs on a large platter. Drizzle the dressing across the top or serve on the side.

NOTE *To prepare ahead:* Place all the ingredients in separate bags and assemble this at work for a fresh-tasting lunch.

VARIATIONS

+ Try Everyone's Favorite Italian Dressing (page 169) for a different flavor.

+ Add 2 cups (370 g) of cooked quinoa for some hearty grain texture.

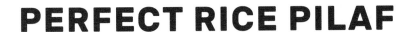
PERFECT RICE PILAF

This is the perfect side dish for any low-FODMAP meal. Rice pilaf is a staple in my house, and it goes well for both weeknights and entertaining. FODMAP fact: Rice is naturally low-FODMAP, so you can enjoy up to 1 cup (190 g) cooked rice for one serving. Try this rice as a base for any stir-fry, serve it cold in a salad, or just eat it plain with a little soy sauce. So good.

Heat the stock in a large saucepan with a lid or in a Dutch oven. Meanwhile, place a large skillet over medium-high heat. Add the olive oil to coat the bottom of the pan. When the oil is hot, add the uncooked rice. Brown the rice in the pan, stirring occasionally, for a couple of minutes. When the rice has browned, place it into the large saucepan. Bring to a simmer, lower the heat, cover, and cook for 15 to 25 minutes, until the rice is soft. Remove the pan from the heat and let sit for 10 minutes, covered. Stir in the fresh parsley and add salt to taste.

4 cups (960 ml) low-FODMAP vegan stock

2 teaspoons (10 ml) onion-infused olive oil (page 25)

2 cups (380 g) long-grain white rice

½ cup (30 g) chopped fresh parsley

Salt to taste (omit if your stock is highly salted)

VARIATIONS

+ For a nonvegan version, use low-FODMAP chicken stock, homemade (page 167) or store-bought (page 21).

+ Garnish with toasted almond slivers or pine nuts, and sprinkle with freshly grated Parmesan for nonvegans.

+ Substitute 1 cup (185 g) white quinoa for 1 cup (190 g) rice and make it a rice-quinoa medley!

SIMPLE STARTERS AND SIDES

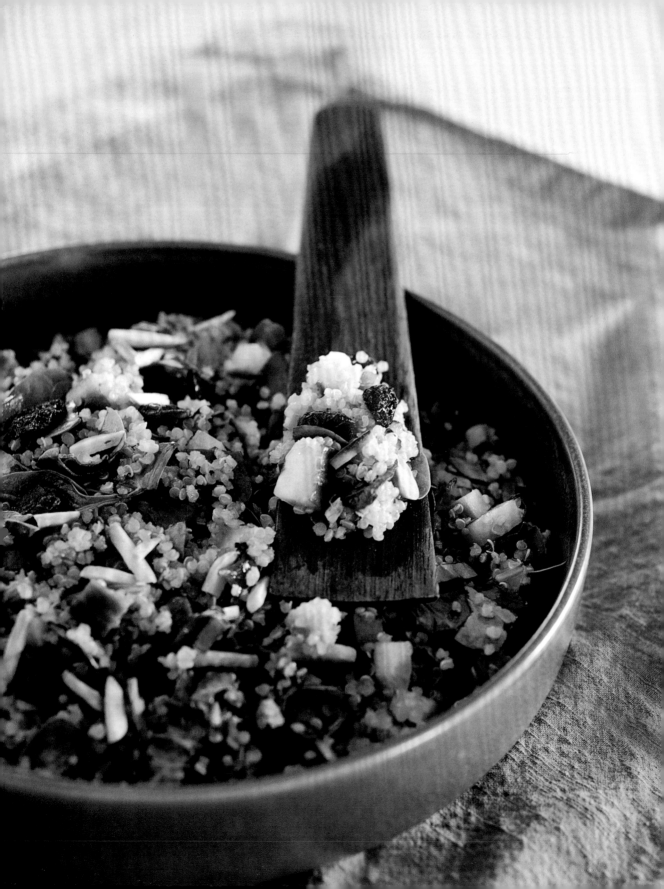

WARM QUINOA AND SPINACH SALAD

This salad is one of my favorites for its simplicity and flavor. Eating the quinoa freshly warm makes it a super-satisfying meal. FODMAP fact: While almonds are often perceived to be high-FODMAP, it depends on their serving size. You can enjoy ½ ounce (12 g) of almonds without issue, but avoid overconsuming them, as this could result in a high-FODMAP serving.

Place the water in a medium saucepan over high heat and add the salt and quinoa. Bring to a boil, then reduce the heat and simmer until the water is absorbed, 10 to 15 minutes. Place the cooked quinoa in a medium serving bowl. Add the spinach and cucumber to the bowl, drizzle with the dressing, and toss to coat. Top with the toasted almond slivers and dried cranberries.

1 cup (240 ml) water

¼ teaspoon salt

½ cup (85 g) white quinoa, rinsed

2 cups (60 g) chopped baby spinach

½ cup (75 g) diced cucumber

3 tablespoons (45 ml) Sensational Soy Maple Dressing (page 159)

¼ cup (24 g) toasted almond slivers (page 40)

2 tablespoons (15 g) dried cranberries

VARIATIONS

+ Try topped with toasted pine nuts or sunflower seeds in place of the almond slivers.

+ This salad also works well with Sesame Ginger Dressing or Marinade (page 164) and Creamy Poppyseed Salad Dressing (page 168)!

SIMPLE STARTERS AND SIDES

SUMMERTIME SALAD WITH TOASTED PECANS

This salad reminds me of Panera's version that I used to love eating every summer. Try it and you will see it is even better with fresh fruits. FODMAP fact: Red grapes have only trace FODMAPs, so you can enjoy this fruit freely.

½ cup (85 g) sliced fresh strawberries

¼ cup (38 g) fresh blueberries

1 cup (165 g) chunked fresh pineapple

¼ cup (38 g) sliced red grapes

¾ cup (80 g) toasted pecans, halved or chopped (page 40)

4 to 5 cups (120 to 150 g) butter lettuce, torn or coarsely chopped

4 to 6 tablespoons (60 to 90 ml) low-FODMAP Creamy Poppyseed Salad Dressing (page 168)

Combine the fruits, nuts, and lettuce in a large bowl and toss with the dressing.

VARIATIONS

+ Sprinkle with ¾ cup (112 g) crumbled feta cheese or goat cheese for non-vegans.

+ Try One-Pot Candied Peanuts (page 49) in place of the pecans for an even sweeter crunch.

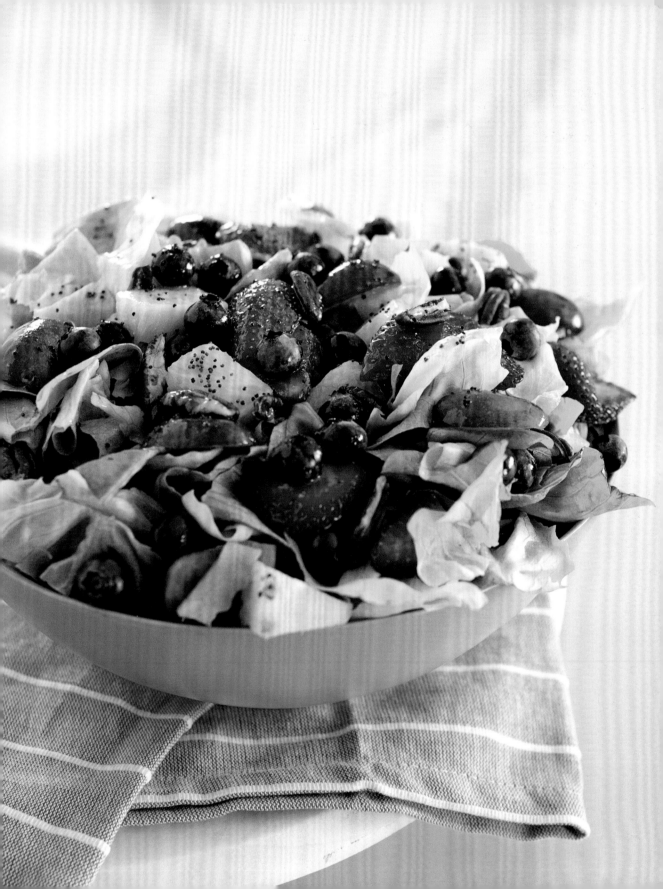

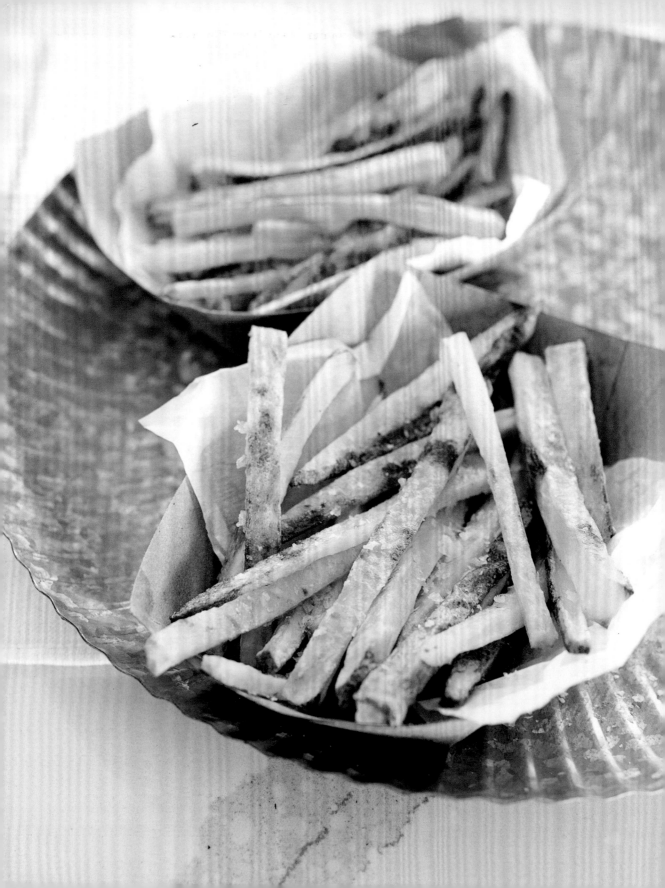

CRISPY BAKED GARLIC FRENCH FRIES

Everyone loves French fries, and these tasty baked garlic fries are delicious and addictive. But don't feel guilty about enjoying them! One medium potato provides 5 g of protein, 5 g of fiber, more potassium than a banana, and only 160 calories. Plus, potatoes are naturally low in FODMAPs as well as gluten-free.

Preheat the oven to 450°F (230°C or gas mark 8). Line two baking sheets with parchment paper and generously coat with cooking spray.

Chop the potatoes into thin strips. Combine both oils in a small glass or bottle. Spread the chopped potatoes on the prepared baking sheets, then drizzle with 1 tablespoon (15 ml) of the oil mixture and sprinkle with salt. Space the potatoes apart in a single layer to allow them to cook faster. Bake for 10 to 15 minutes, rotating the baking sheets midway through cooking for even browning, then remove from the oven and flip all the fries using tongs or a spatula. Drizzle again with 1 tablespoon (15 ml) of the oil and sprinkle with salt. Bake for another 10 minutes, or until crisped to your preference, remove from the oven, sprinkle again with sea salt, and drizzle with the remaining 2 tablespoons (30 ml) oil.

NOTE Spreading the potatoes out well on the baking sheet ensures they cook evenly and crisp faster.

Cooking spray

1½ pounds (680 g) medium russet potatoes, scrubbed clean and dried (3 or 4 medium potatoes)

2 tablespoons (30 ml) olive oil

2 tablespoons (30 ml) garlic-infused olive oil (page 25), divided

Sea salt to taste

VARIATIONS

+ When finished baking, remove the baking sheets from the oven and dust the fries with ¼ cup (25 g) grated Parmesan in addition to the oil, then return to the oven for 3 to 4 minutes to allow the cheese to melt.

+ Try a mushroom-infused oil or truffle oil for a different flavor.

ASIAN VEGETABLE STIR-FRY

This is a classic recipe that you will make again and again. Easy and delicious stir-fry vegetables go well with everything. FODMAP facts: Broccoli heads are lower in FODMAPs than the entire broccoli with stalk. Chop off the heads and enjoy this delicious and healthy vegetable. Also, ⅓ cup (84 g) canned bamboo shoots and ½ cup (75 g) water chestnuts are one low-FODMAP serving.

1 tablespoon (15 ml) oil

½ cup (40 g) broccoli florets

1 tablespoon (15 ml) water

1 cup (120 g) julienned carrot

½ cup (75 g) sliced water chestnuts (canned)

⅔ cup (168 g) bamboo shoots (canned)

1 teaspoon minced fresh ginger

3 tablespoons (45 ml) tamari (gluten-free soy sauce) or soy sauce

3 tablespoons (45 ml) low-FODMAP vegan stock

1 teaspoon cornstarch

Heat a large pan or wok over medium-high heat and add the oil. Add the broccoli and water and stir-fry for 1 minute, or until the broccoli is bright green. Add the carrots, water chestnuts, bamboo shoots, and ginger; stir-fry for 1 to 2 minutes, or until crisp-tender. In a small bowl, combine the tamari, stock, and cornstarch; mix well to dissolve the cornstarch. Add the sauce to the pan and stir-fry for about 1 minute, until the sauce is slightly thickened.

NOTE This stir-fry is delicious over steamed rice or Perfect Rice Pilaf (page 59).

VARIATIONS

+ Sprinkle with toasted sesame seeds or almond slivers.

+ Top with 1 pound (454 g) of cooked chicken breast, shrimp, or crispy tofu (page 133) for some additional protein.

NIÇOISE SALAD

Did you know this salad originated in the French city of Nice? That is how it got its beautiful name. Niçoise salad is a light, healthy, delicious salad that is packed with protein and nutrition. FODMAP facts: Olives provide amazing taste to this salad and are low-FODMAP in ½-cup (60 g) servings. Green beans are also low-FODMAP in 2½-ounce (75 g) servings.

To make the salad: Boil the potatoes in a pot of water until fork-tender (about 10 minutes). Meanwhile, bring a smaller pot of water to a boil, add the green beans, and cook until green and tender, 2 to 4 minutes (or microwave for 1 to 2 minutes in a covered dish with a small amount of water on the bottom). When the beans are cooked, plunge into ice-cold water and pat dry. Next, drain the potatoes and set aside to cool, then chop into wedges.

To make the dressing: While the potatoes are cooling, prepare the dressing by whisking the lemon juice, mustard, olive oil, maple syrup (if using), and salt in a small bowl until well emulsified. Toss the potatoes with 1 tablespoon (15 ml) of the dressing.

Arrange the dressed potatoes, green beans, eggs, spinach, tomatoes, olives, and tuna on a large platter and drizzle with the remaining 5 to 6 tablespoons (75 to 90 ml) dressing.

NOTE An immersion blender works well to emulsify the dressing.

FOR THE SALAD

4 new potatoes, washed

10 ounces (280 g) green beans

2 hard-boiled eggs, sliced

8 ounces (224 g) baby spinach, torn

2 medium ripe tomatoes, diced

¼ cup (30 g) kalamata olives, pitted

One 5-ounce (140 g) can chunk white or light tuna, drained

FOR THE DRESSING

1 tablespoon (15 ml) freshly squeezed lemon juice

1 tablespoon (11 g) Dijon mustard

4 tablespoons (60 ml) olive oil

1 tablespoon (15 ml) maple syrup (optional)

Salt to taste

VARIATION

+ Try seared ahi tuna rather than canned for an upscale version.

SIMPLE STARTERS AND SIDES

CURRIED CHICKPEA SALAD

This creamy chickpea salad gets its amazing flavors from the curry, almonds, and grapes. Although it is suitable for vegans, my meat-loving husband gobbles this up. Serve it with crackers or put it in a lettuce cup! FODMAP facts: Grapes are one of the fruits that do not contain FODMAPs, so you can enjoy as much as you wish. But be aware, drying grapes into raisins changes that amount. Raisins are low-FODMAP in servings of 1 tablespoon (13 g).

6 ounces (168 g) extra-firm tofu, drained

1 tablespoon (15 ml) tamari (gluten-free soy sauce) or soy sauce

One 15-ounce (420 g) can chickpeas, drained and rinsed

5 tablespoons (75 g) vegan mayonnaise (see Note) or full-fat mayonnaise (for non-vegans)

1 teaspoon yellow curry powder (no added onion, garlic)

Salt and pepper to taste

¾ cup (112 g) red grapes, cut in half

2 tablespoons (6 g) chopped chives

¼ cup (25 g) chopped toasted almonds (page 40)

Preheat the oven to 350°F (180°C or gas mark 4). Line a baking sheet with foil. Place the tofu on the prepared baking sheet and drizzle with the tamari. Allow to sit for 5 minutes, turning once. Place the tofu in the oven and roast for 15 minutes. Meanwhile, add the chickpeas to a large bowl and mash them roughly with a potato masher or a fork. Add the mayonnaise, curry powder, salt, and pepper and stir to combine.

When the tofu is ready, allow it to cool for about 5 minutes on the pan, then crumble the tofu with your hands and add it to the chickpea mixture. Add the grapes, chives, and almonds and stir together. Serve immediately, or refrigerate until ready to eat.

NOTE Although vegan mayonnaise has not been formally tested for FODMAPs, there are three brands that are gluten-free and contain ingredients that appear to be low-FODMAP: JUST Mayo, Vegenaise, and Best Foods/Hellmann's Vegan.

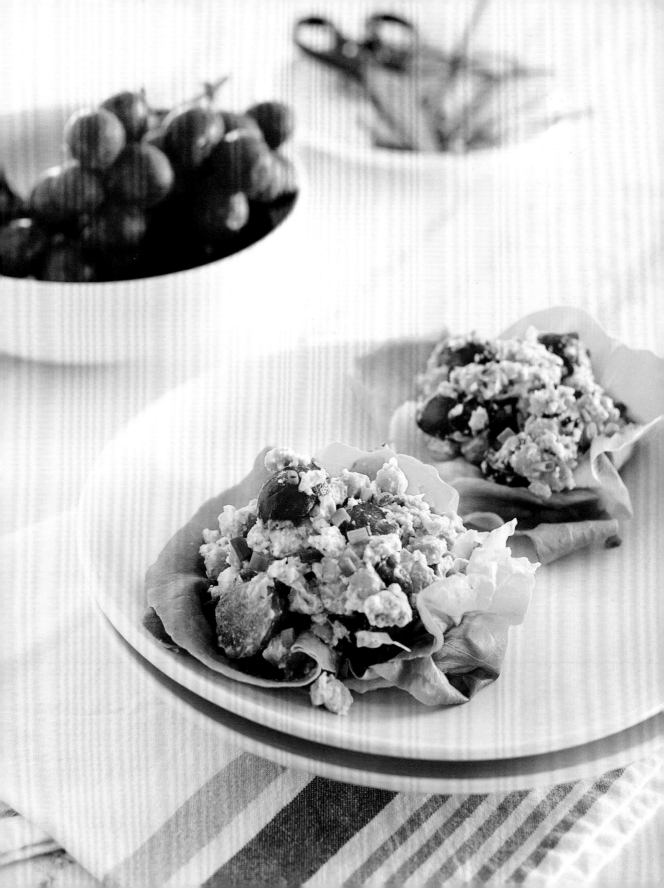

LEMON ROSEMARY NEW POTATOES

My mother used to make new potatoes every summer when they came into season. I have always loved their smooth texture, small size, and sweet flavor. FODMAP fact: Because butter is naturally high in fat, it contains few carbohydrates and is low in lactose levels.

12 new potatoes or small red potatoes (about 1 pound [455 g])

¼ cup (56 g) unsalted butter or vegan margarine

3 sprigs fresh rosemary, broken into pieces, divided

3 tablespoons (45 ml) freshly squeezed lemon juice (about ¾ medium lemon)

1 teaspoon grated lemon zest

Salt and pepper to taste

Place the potatoes in a large saucepan and add enough water to cover them. Bring to a boil over high heat. Lower the heat, cover, and cook for 15 to 20 minutes, or until tender.

Meanwhile, in a small saucepan, melt the butter over medium-low heat. Stir in 2 sprigs of the rosemary and let it infuse the butter for 2 to 3 minutes. Then add the lemon juice and lemon zest and stir to combine. Set aside.

When the potatoes are cooked, drain them and place in a large serving bowl. Sprinkle liberally with salt and pepper. Pour the butter mixture over the potatoes; toss gently to coat. Garnish with the remaining sprig of fresh rosemary.

NOTE Watch the butter closely when cooking to ensure it doesn't burn, as butter has a lower smoke point than other oils.

VARIATION

+ Drizzle some garlic-infused olive oil (page 25) over the potatoes for a little garlic flavor.

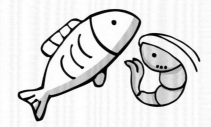

4

HEALTHY FISH AND SHELLFISH

You will love these simple and delicious fish and shellfish recipes. I recommend fish or shellfish two or three times a week for the healthy nutrients that they provide.

BROILED SALMON WITH MAPLE LEMON GLAZE

This salmon recipe is absolutely delicious, super healthy, easy to prep, and effortless to clean up. I love to use freshly squeezed lemon juice to give the best flavor and ensure the recipe is low-FODMAP. FODMAP fact: While apples are considered high-FODMAP, apple cider vinegar is low-FODMAP in a serving size of up to 2 tablespoons (30 ml).

2 tablespoons (30 ml) freshly squeezed lemon juice (about ½ medium lemon)

2 tablespoons (30 ml) pure maple syrup

1 tablespoon (15 ml) apple cider vinegar

1 tablespoon (15 ml) olive oil or other preferred oil

Four 6-ounce (168 g) salmon fillets (skin on or off per your preference)

Salt and ground pepper to taste

Preheat the oven to broil and place the oven rack in the middle position. Combine the lemon juice, maple syrup, apple cider vinegar, and oil in a large resealable plastic bag. Place the salmon in the bag, seal, and refrigerate for 10 minutes, turning the bag once after about 5 minutes. After 10 minutes, remove the salmon from the bag, reserving the marinade. Place the marinade in a microwave-safe bowl and microwave on high for 1 minute (the mixture will be bubbling).

Place a large oven-safe skillet (cast iron works well) over medium-high heat. Place the salmon in the pan, skin side down (if using salmon with skin). Cook for 3 minutes and then flip the salmon and brush the marinade evenly over each fillet. Cook for another 3 minutes and flip again, then brush the marinade over each fillet again. Place under the broiler skin side down for 3 minutes, or until the desired degree of doneness (I recommend medium-rare). Season with salt and pepper to taste.

TIP If you don't have apple cider vinegar, you can substitute a similar amount of extra lemon juice.

VARIATION

+ Try the recipe with freshly squeezed orange juice for a different flavor!

ONE-PAN TILAPIA WITH LEMON, GARLIC, AND CAPERS

You will love this light and satisfying tilapia dinner. The capers and garlic provide savory notes, while the lemon adds zest to the fish. Squeezing your lemon juice fresh tastes far superior and ensures a low-FODMAP product.

In a large nonstick pan, heat both oils over medium heat. Add the tilapia and season with salt and pepper. Cook for 3 to 4 minutes, until the bottom of the fish is brown. Turn the fillets and pour the lemon juice on top. Sprinkle with more salt and pepper and spoon the capers over the fish. Cook for another 3 to 4 minutes. Remove from the pan and serve hot, garnished with sliced lemon, if desired.

1 tablespoon (15 ml) olive oil

1 tablespoon (15 ml) garlic-infused olive oil (page 25)

Four 4- to 5-ounce (112 to 140 g) tilapia fillets, patted dry

Salt and pepper to taste

3 tablespoons (45 ml) freshly squeezed lemon juice (about ¾ medium lemon)

1 tablespoon (9 g) capers, drained

Lemon slices, for garnish (optional)

VARIATION

✦ Add 2 to 3 tablespoons (8 to 12 g) chopped fresh dill instead of the capers for a different flavor.

   Yield: 4 servings   **Prep time:** 18 minutes   **Cook time:** 7 minutes

SWEET AND SAVORY SHRIMP

Shrimp are one of my favorite foods, and this recipe is simple and delicious. The Dijon and maple marinade creates a sweet and savory flavor your whole family will enjoy.

In a large bowl, combine the mustard, maple syrup, and tamari. Add the shrimp to the bowl and stir to coat with the marinade. Let sit, covered, in the refrigerator for 15 minutes, turning once.

   Heat the oil in a large skillet over medium heat, and then add the shrimp and sauce to the skillet. Sauté for 3 to 5 minutes, until the shrimp are cooked through (you want them to be just turned pink). Serve immediately over steamed rice.

¼ cup (45 g) Dijon mustard

2 tablespoons (30 ml) maple syrup

2 tablespoons (30 ml) tamari (gluten-free soy sauce) or soy sauce

1 pound (455 g) large raw shrimp, peeled and deveined (tails on or off, per your preference)

1 tablespoon (15 ml) olive oil

VARIATION

✦ Try it with scallops instead of shrimp!

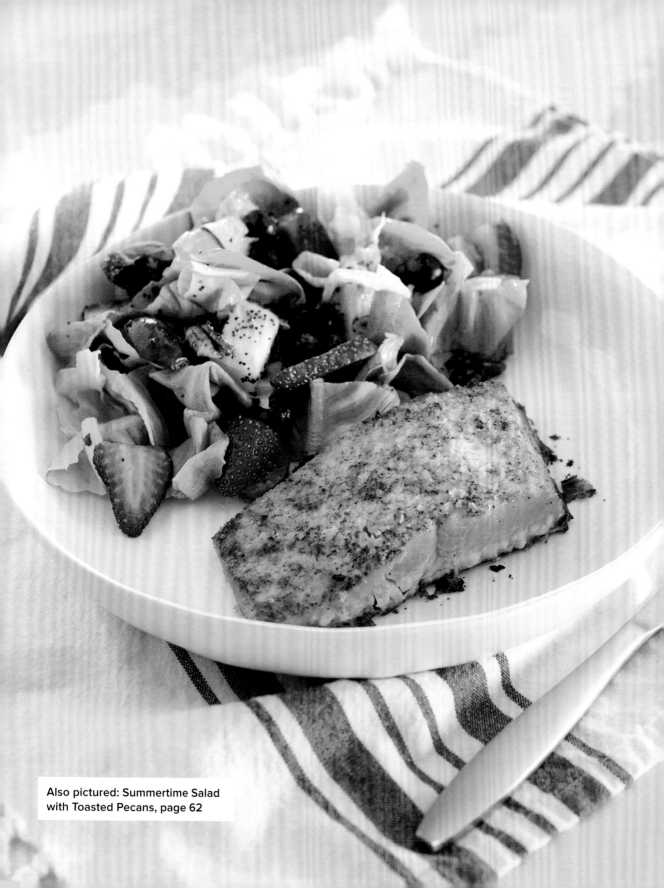

Also pictured: Summertime Salad with Toasted Pecans, page 62

DIJON-CRUSTED SALMON

Dijon-crusted salmon is a classic crowd-pleaser. The mustard gives the salmon a delicious flavor, while the breadcrumbs add welcome texture. You will use this recipe again and again. FODMAP fact: Dijon mustard is a great pantry staple that I use in many recipes. It is low-FODMAP in heaping 1-tablespoon (23 g) servings.

Preheat the oven to 350°F (180°C or gas mark 4) and place the rack in the center of the oven. Line a rectangular baking pan large enough for your salmon pieces with aluminum foil and coat with cooking spray.

Place the salmon fillets in the prepared baking pan, skin side down (if you have salmon with skin), and sprinkle with salt and pepper. Brush the Dijon mustard over the salmon and sprinkle the breadcrumbs on top. Drizzle with the olive oil. Bake for 15 to 20 minutes, or until the salmon is done to your preference (you should be able to flake it slightly with a fork). Let the salmon rest for 5 minutes before serving.

NOTE Lining your pan with foil makes cleanup a breeze!

Cooking spray

Four 4-ounce (112 g) salmon fillets (skin on or off per your preference)

Salt and pepper to taste

2 tablespoons (22 g) Dijon mustard

2 tablespoons (14 g) gluten-free low-FODMAP breadcrumbs

1 tablespoon (15 ml) olive oil

VARIATIONS

+ For a sweeter version, add 1 tablespoon (15 ml) of maple syrup to the Dijon mustard.

+ Try garlic-infused olive oil (page 25) instead of plain olive oil to add some garlic flavor.

HEALTHY FISH AND SHELLFISH

SAUTÉED TILAPIA WITH CHERRY TOMATOES AND OLIVES

This one-pan meal is a snap for any weeknight. Juicy cherry tomatoes, salty olives, and fresh parsley give amazing taste to the fish. Tilapia is one of the most commonly consumed fish in the United States and is also one of the most inexpensive. FODMAP fact: A ½ cup (60 g) of olives is one low-FODMAP serving.

3 tablespoons (45 ml) olive oil

Four 5-ounce (140 g) tilapia fillets, patted dry

Salt and pepper to taste

2 cups (300 g) cherry tomatoes, halved

½ cup (60 g) pitted kalamata olives, halved

½ cup (30 g) chopped fresh parsley

1 tablespoon (15 ml) freshly squeezed lemon juice

Heat the oil in a large skillet over medium-high heat. Add the fish fillets and season with salt and pepper. Cook the fish for about 3 minutes, then turn and cook for another 3 minutes, or until cooked through. Transfer the fish to a covered plate to keep warm.

To the skillet, add the tomatoes, olives, and parsley and cook until soft, 2 to 3 minutes. Add the lemon juice and season with salt and pepper. Remove from heat. Place the fish on a serving plate and pour the sauce over the fish.

VARIATIONS

+ This recipe works great with most fish and shellfish. Try it with shrimp, cod, or scallops.

+ You can substitute canned black olives for the kalamata olives, if necessary.

+ Try infused olive oil (garlic, onion, or basil, see page 25) in place of the olive oil for a different flavor.

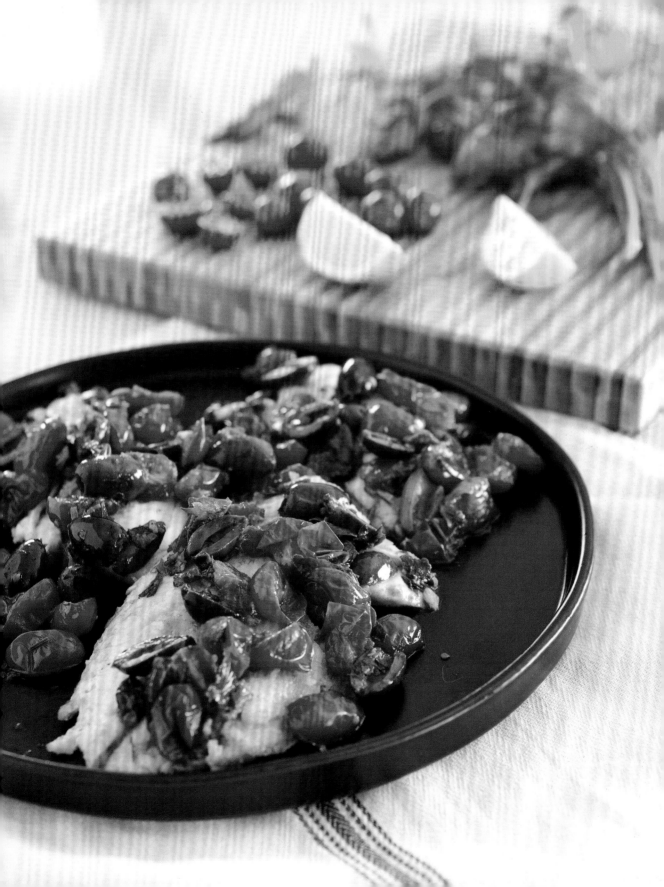

BROILED LEMON PEPPER COD ON PARCHMENT

This cod broiled on parchment paper is so easy and so good. You can enjoy a simple cleanup and have the health benefits of broiled fish. The flavorful oils of lemon are concentrated in the peel, so adding lemon zest gives this dish fantastic lemon flavor.

1 medium lemon

1 tablespoon (15 ml) garlic-infused olive oil (page 25)

½ teaspoon paprika

½ teaspoon salt

½ teaspoon pepper

Four 4-ounce (112 g) cod fillets, patted dry

Preheat the broiler to high and place the rack in the center of the oven. Line a broiler-safe pan with parchment paper.

Zest the lemon into a small bowl, then add the oil, paprika, salt, and pepper and stir to combine. Slice the zested lemon into thin slices. Place the cod fillets on the prepared pan and brush the lemon zest/seasoning mixture on the fish. Place the lemon slices around the cod on the pan. Broil, uncovered, for 4 to 7 minutes, depending on the thickness of the fillets, until the fish flakes easily with a fork. Serve with the cooked lemon slices on top of the fish fillets.

NOTE Do not substitute lemon pepper spice blends, because you won't have the same results.

TIP If you prefer to use your barbecue grill, preheat the grill to high, wrap the fish in foil or use a grill-safe pan, and place on the hot grill for the same length of time.

VARIATION

+ This recipe is delicious with red snapper or flounder fillets instead.

SEARED SCALLOPS WITH BABY SPINACH

Seared scallops are a nutritious treat, and making them at home is much more affordable than going out to a restaurant. Scallops contain 17 grams of protein per 90 calories, plus iron and selenium, and they are naturally low fat. This meal combines the delicious flavor of scallops with delicate sautéed spinach. Bet you can't wait to try it!

Heat the infused oil in a large skillet over medium heat. Add the spinach and cook until wilted, 3 to 5 minutes. The spinach will shrink dramatically as it cooks. Squeeze half the lemon over the spinach and season liberally with salt. Remove the spinach from the pan and set it aside in a covered dish to keep warm. If you have extra lemon juice collected in the pan, pour it over the spinach or discard.

Add the olive oil to the pan and heat again over medium heat. Place the scallops in the pan and cook each side for 2 to 3 minutes (do not overcook). Squeeze the remaining lemon half over the scallops and season with salt and pepper. Remove the pan from the heat. Divide the spinach among serving plates, then lay the scallops on the bed of spinach.

NOTE I prefer cast-iron skillets to sear my scallops; these pans are naturally nonstick and chemical free, last forever, and add some extra iron to your food.

1 tablespoon (15 ml) garlic-infused olive oil (page 25)

10 ounces (280 g) baby spinach, rinsed and dried

1 medium lemon, halved, divided

Salt and pepper to taste

1 tablespoon (15 g) olive oil

1¼ pounds (560 g) scallops, rinsed and patted dry

VARIATION
+ Substitute shrimp, tilapia, or another fish for the scallops.

HEALTHY FISH AND SHELLFISH

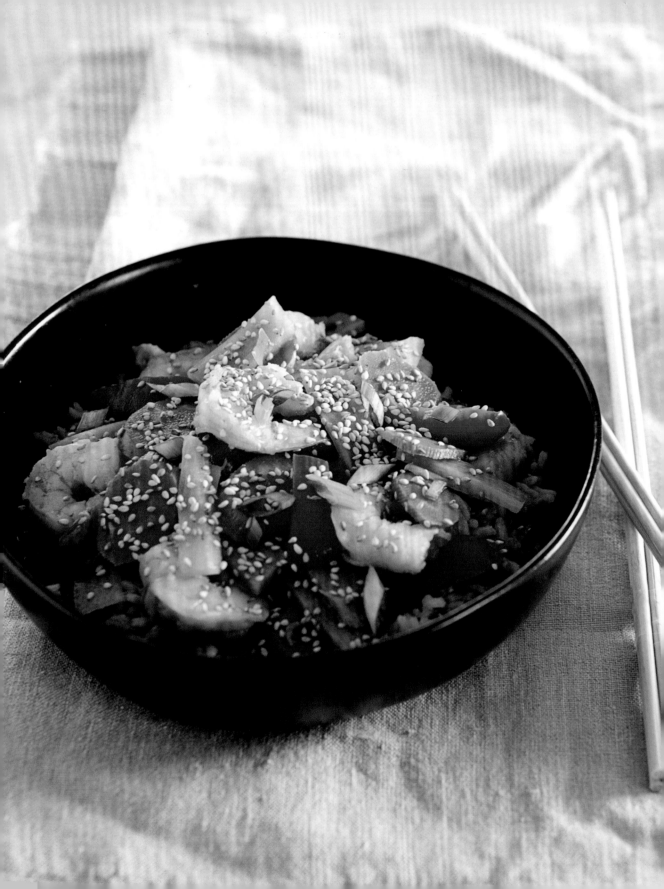

AMAZING SHRIMP STIR-FRY

Shrimp stir-fry is a winner at every table. Shrimp are the most popular seafood in the United States and are low in calories but high in protein. Plus, they taste amazing. FODMAP fact: A ⅓ cup (84 g) of bamboo shoots is one low-FODMAP serving; this vegetable is packed with potassium and a good source of fiber.

Heat 1 tablespoon (15 ml) of the infused oil in a large pan or wok over medium-high heat. Add the shrimp and stir-fry until just turning pink, 4 to 5 minutes, then transfer them to a plate and cover to keep warm.

Heat the remaining 1 tablespoon (15 ml) infused oil in the pan over medium-high heat. Add the ginger, bell pepper, carrots, and bamboo shoots; cook and stir for 3 minutes. Add the tamari, rice vinegar, brown sugar, and sesame oil and stir to combine. Return the shrimp to the pan and toss it all gently to coat. Season with salt and pepper to taste. Serve over steamed rice.

2 tablespoons (30 ml) garlic-infused olive oil (page 25), divided

1 pound (455 g) raw shrimp, peeled (tails on or off, per your preference)

2 teaspoons (6 g) grated fresh ginger

1 medium red bell pepper, cored, seeded, and cut into 1-inch (2.5 cm) pieces

2 medium carrots, cut into ¼-inch (6 mm) coins

1 cup (252 g) canned bamboo shoots, drained

2 tablespoons (30 ml) tamari (gluten-free soy sauce) or soy sauce

2 tablespoons (30 ml) rice vinegar (not seasoned rice vinegar, as that has sugar added)

1 tablespoon (15 g) packed brown sugar

1 teaspoon toasted sesame oil

Salt and pepper to taste

VARIATIONS

+ Sprinkle toasted sesame seeds or scallion tips over the top for garnish.

+ Substitute tofu for the shrimp and you have a delicious vegan stir-fry option instead.

HEALTHY FISH AND SHELLFISH

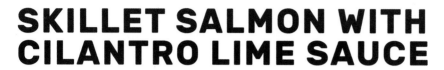
SKILLET SALMON WITH CILANTRO LIME SAUCE

Rich and flavorful salmon with a fresh and light cilantro lime sauce is an impressive meal in less than 20 minutes. It will be a hit in your home! I love to use the cilantro sauce for my Baja fish tacos (page 86) as well.

FOR THE CILANTRO LIME SAUCE

½ cup (120 g) lactose-free sour cream or lactose-free yogurt

2 tablespoons (8 g) green scallion tips

½ cup (8 g) packed cilantro leaves

1½ tablespoons (23 ml) freshly squeezed lime juice (1 medium lime)

1 teaspoon garlic-infused olive oil (page 25)

FOR THE SALMON

1 teaspoon ground cumin

½ teaspoon ground coriander

Pinch of cayenne pepper

½ teaspoon salt, plus more to taste

½ teaspoon freshly ground black pepper, plus more to taste

Four 6-ounce (168 g) salmon fillets, about 1 inch (2.5 cm) thick (skin on or off, per your preference), patted dry

1 tablespoon (15 ml) olive oil

To make the cilantro lime sauce: Place all the sauce ingredients in a large glass and use an immersion blender to process until the cilantro is in very small pieces, or use a stand blender instead. Cover and place in the refrigerator until ready to serve.

To make the salmon: In a small bowl, whisk together the cumin, coriander, cayenne, salt, and pepper. Season both sides of the salmon fillets with the spice blend. Heat the oil in a large cast-iron skillet over medium-high heat. Add the salmon (if skin on, put skin side down first). Cook for about 4 minutes, without moving, until golden brown on the bottom. Flip and cook the salmon on the other side until cooked through, 2 to 3 minutes longer (thicker fillets will take longer). Divide the salmon among serving plates and drizzle with the cilantro lime sauce.

NOTE This salmon is delicious with Perfect Rice Pilaf (page 59) or baked potatoes and steamed broccoli heads.

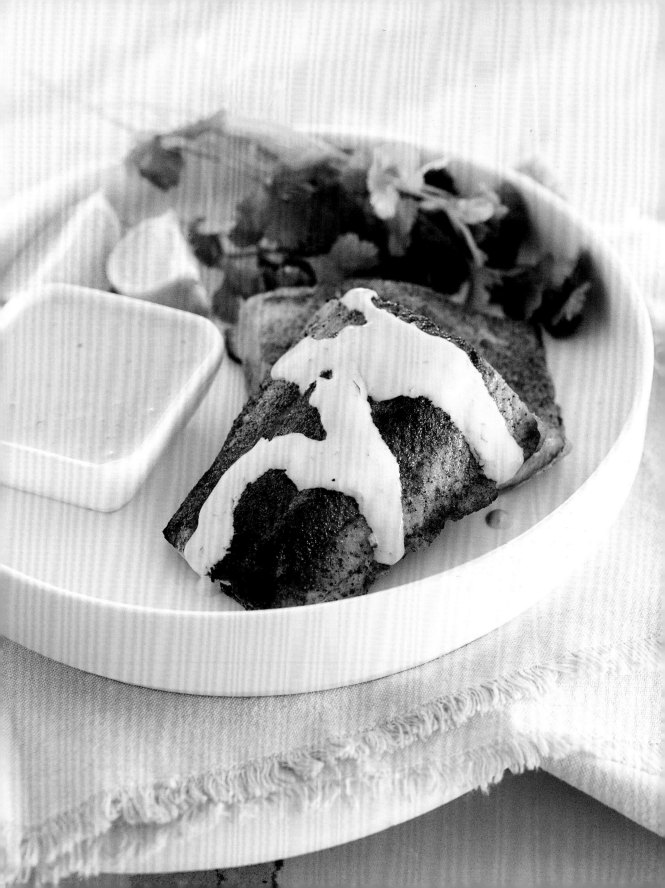

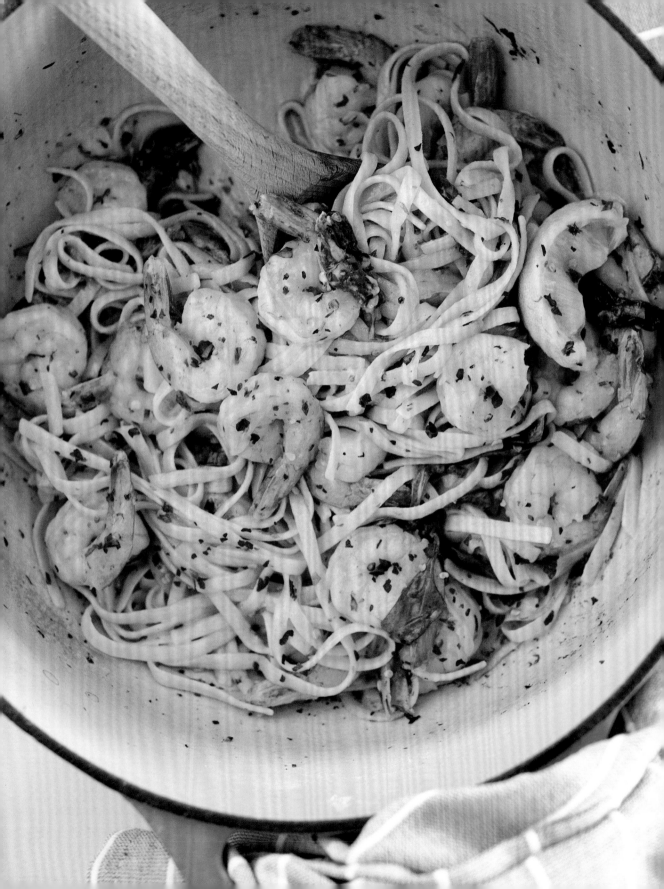

ONE-POT GARLIC SHRIMP PASTA

Amazing flavor without FODMAPs. Garlic-infused olive oil is the star of this recipe! You will taste the flavors of your favorite Italian restaurant, and no one will know how easy this meal was. FODMAP fact: A generous 1½ cups (75 g) of baby spinach is one low-FODMAP serving.

8 ounces (224 g) gluten-free low-FODMAP linguine or spaghettini

2 tablespoons (30 ml) garlic-infused olive oil (page 25), divided

6 tablespoons (84 g) unsalted butter, divided

1 teaspoon red pepper flakes (optional)

1¼ pounds (560 g) large raw shrimp, peeled and deveined (tails on or off, per your preference)

Salt and pepper to taste

1 teaspoon low-FODMAP Italian seasoning, homemade (page 49) or store-bought

4 cups (200 g) baby spinach

½ cup (50 g) grated Parmesan cheese

2 tablespoons (8 g) chopped fresh parsley

1 tablespoon (15 ml) freshly squeezed lemon juice

Bring a large pot of water to a boil over medium-high heat, add the pasta, and cook following package instructions until al dente. Drain and toss with 1 tablespoon (15 ml) of the infused oil. Set aside.

Using the same pot, heat the remaining 1 tablespoon (15 ml) of olive oil and 2 tablespoons (28 g) of the butter. Add the red pepper flakes, if using, and cook until fragrant, 1 to 2 minutes. Add the shrimp, season with salt and pepper, and cook until the shrimp start to turn pink, 4 to 5 minutes. Add the Italian seasoning and spinach and cook until wilted, 3 to 5 minutes.

Add the pasta back to the pot along with the remaining 4 tablespoons (56 g) butter, Parmesan, and parsley. Stir until mixed and the butter is melted. Add the lemon juice just before serving. Best served immediately.

TIP If you prefer an even faster prep, use two pots and cook the pasta at the same time as the shrimp.

THE BEST BAJA FISH TACOS

It doesn't have to be Tuesday for you to love these tacos! This is a healthy, fresh, and delicious meal that combines the flavors of fish, lime, spices, and crunchy cabbage. I love it dipped in my Restaurant-Style Salsa (page 161) or drizzled with my Cilantro Lime Sauce (page 82). FODMAP fact: Avocados can be enjoyed on a low-FODMAP diet, but stick to ⅛ avocado per serving. Even this small amount adds great flavor.

2 cups (180 g) thinly sliced green cabbage

¼ cup (60 g) full-fat mayonnaise

Juice of 1½ limes, divided

¼ cup (24 g) low-FODMAP taco seasoning, homemade (page 100) or store-bought (see Note)

1 pound (455 g) mahi-mahi fish fillets, cut into 1-inch (2.5 cm) pieces

1 tablespoon (15 ml) canola oil

Eight 6-inch (15 cm) soft corn tortillas or gluten-free low-FODMAP soft flour tortillas

½ avocado, sliced into 8 portions

½ cup (120 ml) Restaurant-Style Salsa (page 160)

Chopped cilantro, for serving (optional)

Lime wedges, for serving

In a large bowl, toss cabbage with the mayonnaise and juice from ½ lime. Set aside.

In a freezer bag, combine the remaining juice from 1 lime and the taco seasoning. Shake to combine. Add the fish fillets to the bag and turn to coat. Place the bag in the refrigerator for 10 minutes, turning once after 5 minutes. Drain the fish and discard the marinade.

Heat the oil in a large skillet over medium-high heat. Add the fish pieces and cook for 3 to 4 minutes, then flip and cook for 3 to 4 minutes longer, until cooked through. Remove from the heat.

If desired, warm the tortillas in the microwave or in a clean skillet. Lay the tortillas on a large serving platter and divide the fish, cabbage slaw, avocado, and salsa equally among them. Sprinkle with the cilantro and served with the lime wedges.

NOTE Low-FODMAP taco seasonings are available at online vendors (page 21), or make your own using the recipe on page 100. Beware of store-bought taco blends because they often contain onion and garlic.

VARIATION

+ Try this with red (purple) cabbage or combine red and green for more color. Red cabbage is low-FODMAP in ¾-cup (75 g) servings.

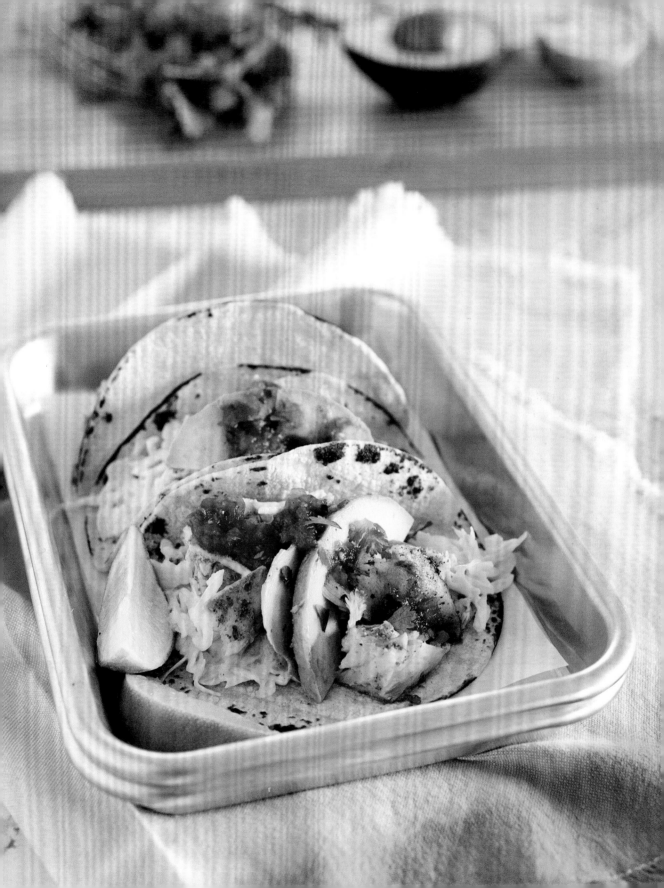

TASTY TUNA SALAD

This is the best tuna salad recipe I have tried. It is creamy and so delicious. I love it on a low-FODMAP roll with sliced tomatoes and lettuce, or as a "tuna melt" (see Tip). FODMAP fact: Although celery is often perceived as a high-FODMAP food, half a medium stalk (10 g) is safe to consume. That is the perfect amount to provide great crunch and flavor for this tuna salad!

Three 5-ounce (140 g) cans white or light albacore tuna, drained

½ cup (120 g) mayonnaise

2 teaspoons (10 ml) freshly squeezed lemon juice

1 teaspoon yellow mustard or Dijon mustard

½ teaspoon black pepper

1 tablespoon (4 g) chopped chives or green scallion tips

½ medium celery stalk (10 g), minced

Place the tuna in a medium bowl and mince it well with a fork until you have fine crumbs. Add the mayonnaise, lemon juice, mustard, pepper, chives, and celery and stir to combine. Store in the refrigerator.

NOTE This tuna salad tastes great made a day ahead.

TIP *Bonus recipe!* To make a tuna melt: Place the desired bread on a microwave- or oven-safe plate and spread with the tuna salad. Place 1½ ounces (40 g) of your preferred cheese (Cheddar, mozzarella, Colby, and Swiss work well) over the tuna. Microwave on high for 30 seconds to 1 minute, or place in a toaster oven on broil and cook until the cheese is bubbly.

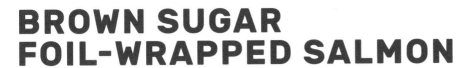
BROWN SUGAR FOIL-WRAPPED SALMON

This is my favorite way to make salmon. The brown sugar glazes the salmon with amazing sweetness, while the foil wrapping locks in moisture and keeps the fish tender. Plus, you just toss the foil in the trash when you're done! So simple. Try it in the oven *or* grill.

Preheat a grill to medium-high or the oven to 375°F (190°C or gas mark 5).

Combine the sugar, oils, tamari, lemon juice, pepper, and salt in a large resealable bag and shake to blend. Add the salmon fillets and turn to coat the fish evenly. Place the bagged salmon in the refrigerator for 10 minutes, turning the bag once. Remove the salmon from the fridge.

Take one or more large pieces of aluminum foil and lay each piece of salmon on its own foil, skin side down. Spoon the remaining marinade from the bag over the salmon pieces. Seal the salmon tightly in the foil and place the packets over indirect heat on the grill or on a baking sheet in the oven. Cook for about 15 minutes. When done, the fish should flake easily with a fork (you can peek at one of the pieces if necessary). Remove the packets from the heat and let rest for 5 minutes before opening (be careful of hot steam!).

NOTE Salmon will continue cooking after you remove it from the heat. It is best to allow it to rest for 5 minutes before serving, similar to steak or other meats.

¼ cup (60 g) brown sugar

3 tablespoons (45 ml) olive oil

1 tablespoon (15 ml) garlic-infused olive oil (page 25)

¼ cup (60 ml) tamari (gluten-free soy sauce) or soy sauce

¼ cup (60 ml) freshly squeezed lemon juice (1 to 2 lemons)

1 teaspoon freshly ground black pepper

½ teaspoon kosher salt

1¼ pounds salmon (skin on or off, per your preference), either 1 large piece or 4 fillets

VARIATIONS

+ You can make salmon with any marinade you love using this method. Try it with my Bold BBQ Sauce (page 163) or Sesame Ginger Dressing or Marinade (page 164).

+ Garnish with toasted sesame seeds and fresh lemon or lime slices.

HEALTHY FISH AND SHELLFISH

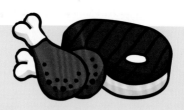

DELICIOUS MEAT AND POULTRY

Your whole family will enjoy these mealtime favorites,
and you will love the easy prep and cleanup!

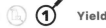
CHICKEN BREASTS WITH ROSEMARY AND ARTICHOKE HEARTS

Artichokes are edible plants that are powerhouses of nutritional benefits. They contain more antioxidants than any other vegetable and are full of fiber. Just 47 calories of artichokes contain 5 grams of fiber, 3 grams of protein, and a plethora of vitamins and minerals. FODMAP fact: One serving of ½ cup (75 g) of canned artichoke hearts is low-FODMAP.

In a large nonstick pan, heat the olive oil and infused oil over medium-high heat. Add the rosemary and let it infuse the oil for 1 to 2 minutes. Add the chicken pieces and sauté until cooked, about 10 minutes. Lower the heat and add the artichokes and lemon juice. Heat the sauce for 2 to 3 minutes, then add salt and pepper to taste. Remove from the heat and serve.

NOTE This meal goes well with steamed quinoa or Perfect Rice Pilaf (page 59).

TIP If you don't have fresh rosemary, then use 1 to 2 tablespoons (3 to 6 g) dried rosemary plus extra to taste.

2 tablespoons (30 ml) olive oil

1 tablespoon (15 ml) garlic-infused olive oil (page 25)

3 tablespoons (5 g) chopped fresh rosemary

3 pounds (1365 g) boneless skinless chicken breasts, cut into 1-inch (2.5 cm) pieces

Two 14-ounce (392 g) cans artichoke hearts, drained and coarsely chopped

¼ cup (60 ml) freshly squeezed lemon juice (about 1 medium lemon)

Salt and ground pepper to taste

ROASTED CHICKEN WITH SPICED MAPLE GLAZE

This is an amazing chicken dinner with a sweet and spicy flavor. Adding cumin and cinnamon gives warm and familiar notes to the tangy mustard glaze. I love using an array of spices in my low-FODMAP cooking, so I never miss the onion and garlic!

Cooking spray

1½ teaspoons paprika

¾ teaspoon ground cinnamon

¾ teaspoon ground cumin

One whole chicken (4 to 5 pounds [1.8 to 2.3 kg]), cut into pieces

3 tablespoons (45 ml) maple syrup

2 tablespoons (28 g) unsalted vegan margarine or butter

1½ tablespoons (16 g) Dijon mustard

Salt and pepper to taste

Preheat the oven to 500°F (250°C or gas mark 10) and place a rack in the upper third of the oven. Line a baking sheet with foil and spray with cooking spray.

In a small bowl, combine the paprika, cinnamon, and cumin. Place the chicken skin side up on the baking sheet and rub the spice mixture evenly over the pieces. Bake for 15 minutes. You don't need to turn the pieces.

Meanwhile, in a microwave-safe bowl or mug, combine the syrup, margarine, and mustard, and heat in 30-second intervals until melted. Stir to combine well.

After 15 minutes, remove the chicken from the oven and brush it with the spiced maple glaze.

Return the chicken to the oven and bake for 5 minutes longer, then remove the chicken a second time, brush with the glaze, and bake for 5 minutes more (the juices should run clear when the chicken is pierced with a knife).

NOTE This chicken is delicious with a baked potato or Perfect Rice Pilaf (page 59).

TIP Buying a whole chicken is often more economical than chicken pieces, but feel free to substitute if you prefer individual thighs or drumsticks for this recipe.

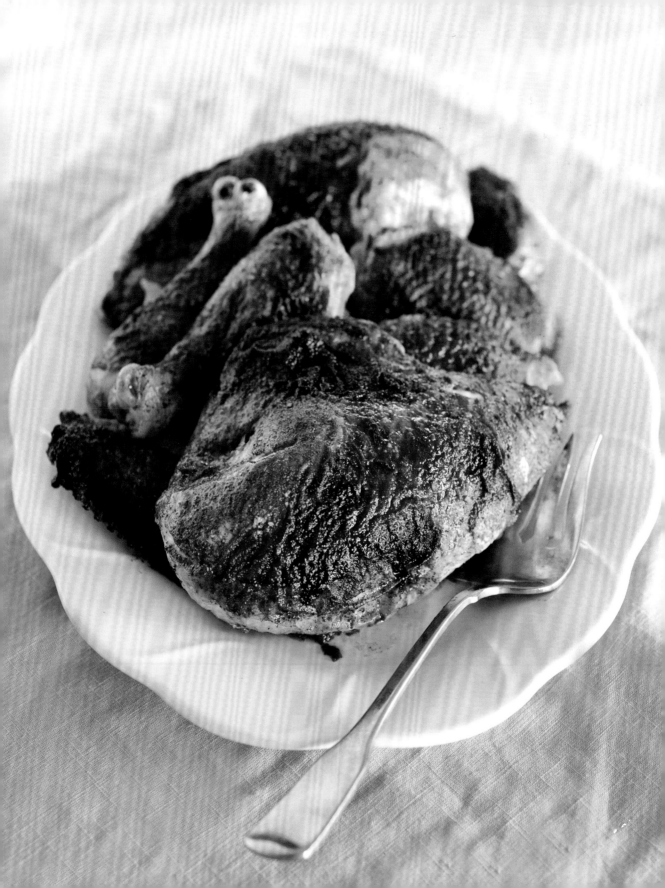

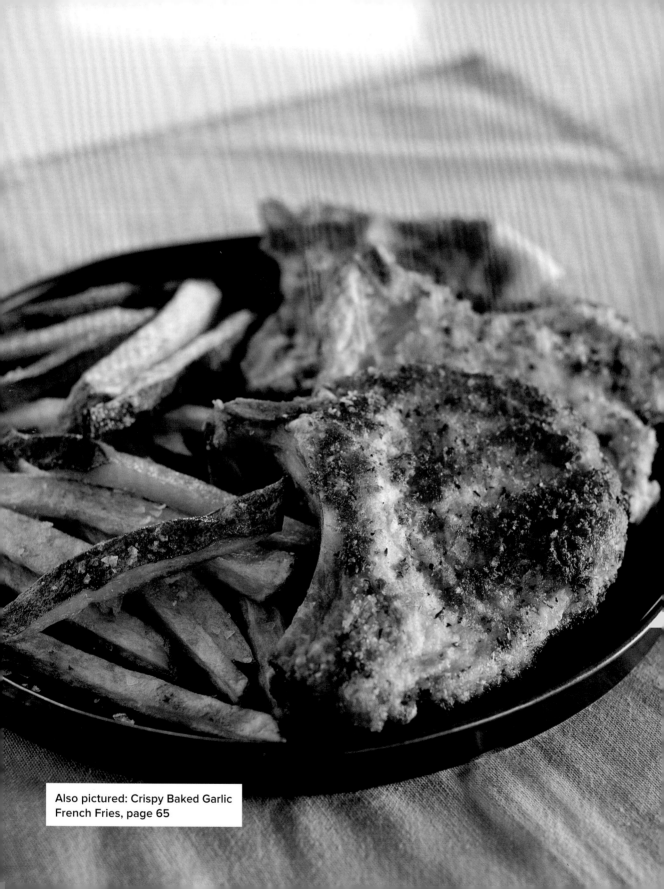

Also pictured: Crispy Baked Garlic French Fries, page 65

CLASSIC BREADED PORK CHOPS

A classic family favorite, these low-FODMAP breaded pork chops are simple to prepare and absolutely delicious. When choosing a suitable low-FODMAP flour, pick one that does not contain ground almonds, chickpeas, or other legumes. Check out my shopping list on page 25 for some options.

Set out three shallow medium bowls. In one bowl, place the low-FODMAP flour. In a second bowl, whisk the eggs with the salt and pepper. In the third bowl, combine the breadcrumbs with the oregano, thyme, and rosemary. Dredge a pork chop in the flour, shaking off the excess, then dip into the eggs and then the breadcrumb mixture. Coat each piece evenly. Set aside on a piece of wax paper or a cutting board. Repeat with the remaining pork chops.

Heat a large skillet over medium heat and add oil to a depth of about 1 inch (2.5 cm). When the oil is hot, add the chops and fry until golden brown and crispy, 3 to 4 minutes on each side.

NOTE Try this meal with steamed carrots and parsnips, Perfect Rice Pilaf (page 59), or Crispy Baked Garlic French Fries (page 65).

TIP Instead of the oregano, thyme, and rosemary, substitute 1 teaspoon low-FODMAP Italian seasoning, homemade (page 49) or store-bought.

⅓ cup (40 g) all-purpose gluten-free low-FODMAP flour

2 eggs

1 teaspoon salt

Freshly ground pepper to taste

½ cup (60 g) gluten-free low-FODMAP breadcrumbs

¼ teaspoon dried oregano

¼ teaspoon dried thyme

¼ teaspoon dried rosemary

4 bone-in pork chops (1½ pounds [680 g]), about ½ inch (1.3 cm) thick, patted dry

Canola oil, for frying

DELICIOUS MEAT AND POULTRY

GRILLED STEAK WITH SOY AND LIME

Steak is the perfect grilling food, and you will love the simplicity of this recipe. Lime provides a hint of citrus that tastes like summer all year-round.

¼ cup (60 ml) tamari (gluten-free soy sauce) or soy sauce

2 tablespoons (30 ml) freshly squeezed lime juice (about 1 lime)

1 tablespoon (15 ml) garlic-infused olive oil (page 25)

1 teaspoon minced fresh ginger

1 tablespoon (15 g) brown sugar

2½ pounds (1138 g) New York strip or sirloin steak, about 1 inch (2.5 cm) thick

Preheat the grill to medium-high.

Place the tamari, lime juice, oil, ginger, and brown sugar in a large resealable bag and shake to combine. Add the steaks and turn to coat. Seal the bag and marinate in the refrigerator for 10 minutes, turning after 5 minutes.

Remove the steaks from the marinade and grill for 8 to 10 minutes, until the desired doneness.

VARIATION

+ Substitute chicken or fish (such as mahi-mahi or tilapia) for the steak.

MEDITERRANEAN CHICKEN WITH OLIVES AND TOMATOES

This meal's flavors are complex and satisfying. Green olives provide great texture, taste, and color.

2 teaspoons (10 ml) garlic-infused olive oil (page 25), divided

1½ pounds (680 g) boneless skinless chicken breasts, cut into 1-inch (2.5 cm) pieces

One 15-ounce (420 g) can diced tomatoes (no added onion, garlic)

½ cup (50 g) pitted green olives, chopped or whole

1 tablespoon (6 g) low-FODMAP Italian seasoning, homemade (page 49) or store-bought

In a large skillet, heat 1 teaspoon (5 ml) of the infused oil over medium-high heat. Add the chicken pieces and sauté until just cooked through, about 6 minutes. Transfer the chicken to a covered plate and set aside. Wipe out the skillet.

Heat the remaining 1 teaspoon (5 ml) infused oil in the skillet, then add the tomatoes, olives, and Italian seasoning. Cook, stirring, until heated through, about 5 minutes. Add the chicken back to the pan and cook until warmed through, spooning the sauce over the chicken.

VARIATION

+ Sprinkle with 1 to 2 tablespoons (9 to 18 g) capers for more Mediterranean flavor.

TANGY TURKEY SLOPPY JOES

This recipe is my twist on a classic Sloppy Joe. I use turkey instead of beef and add a little sweetness to the sauce. It is super tasty and will please even the pickiest eaters. FODMAP fact: While high-fructose corn syrup is high-FODMAP, regular corn syrup is safe to consume. Ketchup is low-FODMAP in ⅓-ounce (13 g) servings (about 2 teaspoons), but choose brands without high-fructose corn syrup.

In a large pan, heat the oil over medium-high heat. Add the ground turkey and cook until browned, 3 to 5 minutes. Drain the excess liquid, leaving the turkey in the pan. Place the pan back over medium heat and add the ketchup, corn syrup, and tamari. Mix together well.

In a small bowl, combine the chicken stock and cornstarch and stir to dissolve the cornstarch. Add the stock mixture to the pan and stir into the turkey mixture. Cook over medium heat until the sauce is thickened, 5 to 8 minutes, adjusting the heat if necessary. Add salt and pepper to taste. Spoon about ⅓ cup (80 g) of the mixture onto each bun and serve hot.

NOTE I like Udi's gluten-free hamburger buns for this meal.

1 tablespoon (15 ml) garlic-infused olive oil (page 25)

1 pound (455 g) ground turkey

¼ cup (60 ml) ketchup

¼ cup (60 ml) light corn syrup

3 tablespoons (45 ml) tamari (gluten-free soy sauce) or soy sauce

½ cup (120 ml) low-FODMAP chicken stock, homemade (page 167) or store-bought (page 21)

3 tablespoons (24 g) cornstarch

Salt and pepper to taste

6 gluten-free low-FODMAP buns

VARIATION

+ Try it with ground beef or chicken instead.

BREADED MINIATURE TURKEY BURGERS

You don't need a bun for these delicious mini turkey burgers. Coating them with breadcrumbs provides a tasty crust that your kids will love. Serve them with Copycat Secret Sauce (page 169) or ketchup.

2 pounds (910 g) ground turkey

½ cup (30 g) minced fresh parsley

1 teaspoon low-FODMAP Italian seasoning, homemade (page 49) or store-bought

½ teaspoon salt

1 tablespoon (15 ml) garlic-infused olive oil (page 25)

2 tablespoons (30 ml) freshly squeezed lemon juice (about ½ medium lemon)

½ cup (60 g) gluten-free low-FODMAP breadcrumbs

2 tablespoons (30 ml) canola oil

In a large bowl, combine the turkey, parsley, seasoning, salt, infused oil, and lemon juice. Mix well with your hands. Form the turkey mixture into 16 miniature patties about 2 inches (5 cm) in diameter. Put the breadcrumbs in a shallow dish. Press the burgers into the breadcrumbs on all sides; set aside.

In a large skillet, heat the canola oil over medium-high heat. Add the patties and cook until cooked through, about 5 minutes per side, depending on thickness (do not overcook, or they will become dry). Serve immediately.

NOTE Try these with my Crispy Baked Garlic French Fries (page 65) and a tossed salad.

VARIATION

+ Try 1 teaspoon yellow curry powder in the turkey mixture for a totally different flavor.

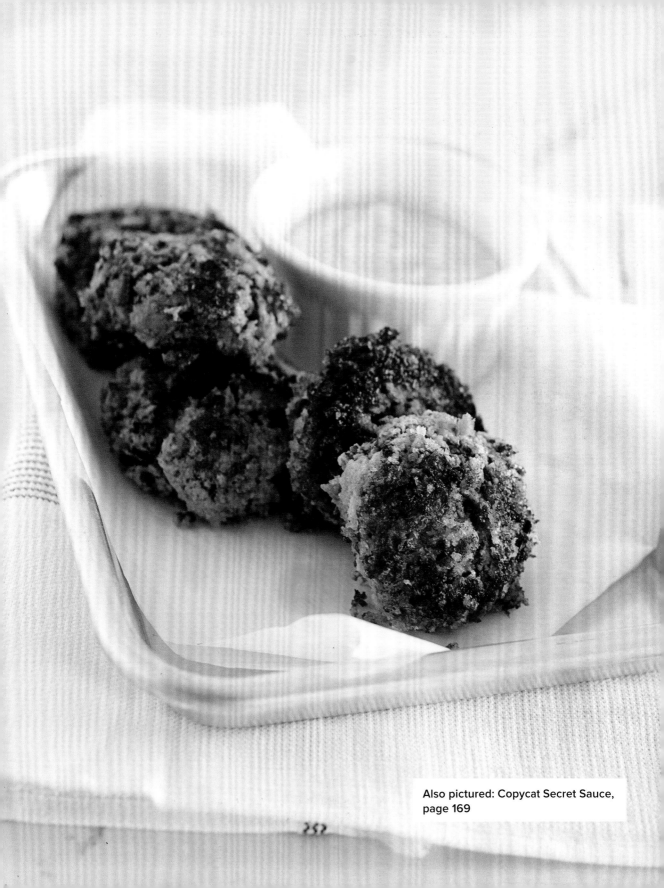

Also pictured: Copycat Secret Sauce, page 169

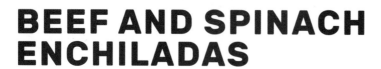
BEEF AND SPINACH ENCHILADAS

Easy, filling, and so good for you, these enchiladas are a favorite at our house. We probably enjoy them two or three times a month. FODMAP fact: Because cheese is naturally low in lactose, you can enjoy this food on the low-FODMAP diet. However, because cheese is high in fat, restrict consumption if it is a trigger for your IBS.

Cooking spray

1½ pounds (680 g) extra-lean ground beef

2 tablespoons (30 ml) olive oil

3 cups (150 g) baby spinach

1 cup (250 g) canned diced tomatoes

2 tablespoons (8 g) low-FODMAP taco seasoning, homemade (see Tip) or store-bought

Salt and pepper to taste

1 cup (120 g) shredded Cheddar cheese, divided

Eight 6-inch (15 cm) soft corn tortillas or gluten-free low-FODMAP soft flour tortillas (see Note on page 45 for more about choosing and preparing tortillas)

Restaurant-Style Salsa (page 160), for serving (optional)

Lactose-free sour cream, for serving (optional)

Preheat the oven to 350°F (180°C or gas mark 4) and spray a 9 by 13-inch (23 x 33 cm) casserole dish with cooking spray.

In a large skillet over medium heat, brown the beef until cooked through, 5 to 10 minutes. Transfer to a covered dish to keep warm. Wipe out the skillet. Add the olive oil to the skillet and sauté the spinach until wilted, about 5 minutes. Drain any excess water from the pan and from the plated beef.

Return the beef to the pan with the spinach and add the tomatoes, seasoning, and salt and pepper to taste. Cook for about 1 minute, then remove from the heat and stir in ¾ cup (90 g) of the cheese. Place the tortillas on a cutting board and divide the beef mixture evenly among them. Roll up the tortillas and place them in the prepared casserole dish. Sprinkle the remaining ¼ cup (30 g) cheese on top. Cover the dish with foil and bake for about 10 minutes, then remove the foil and bake for 5 minutes more, until the cheese is melted and the tortillas are heated through. Serve with salsa and sour cream, if desired.

TIP *Bonus recipe!* If you don't have low-FODMAP taco seasoning, combine 1½ tablespoons (9 g) ancho chile powder and 1½ teaspoons ground cumin.

VARIATION

+ Try this with ground chicken or turkey instead of beef.

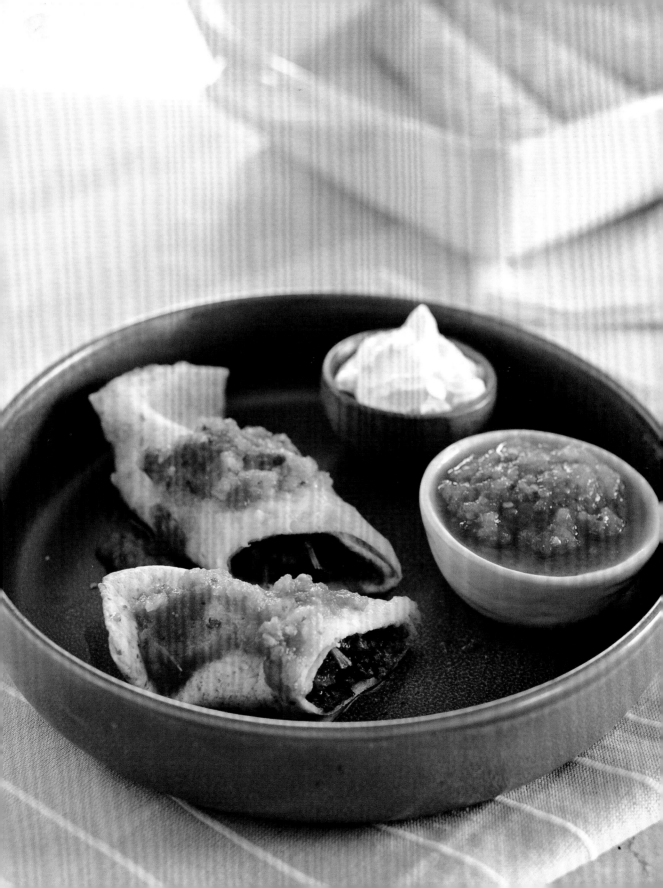

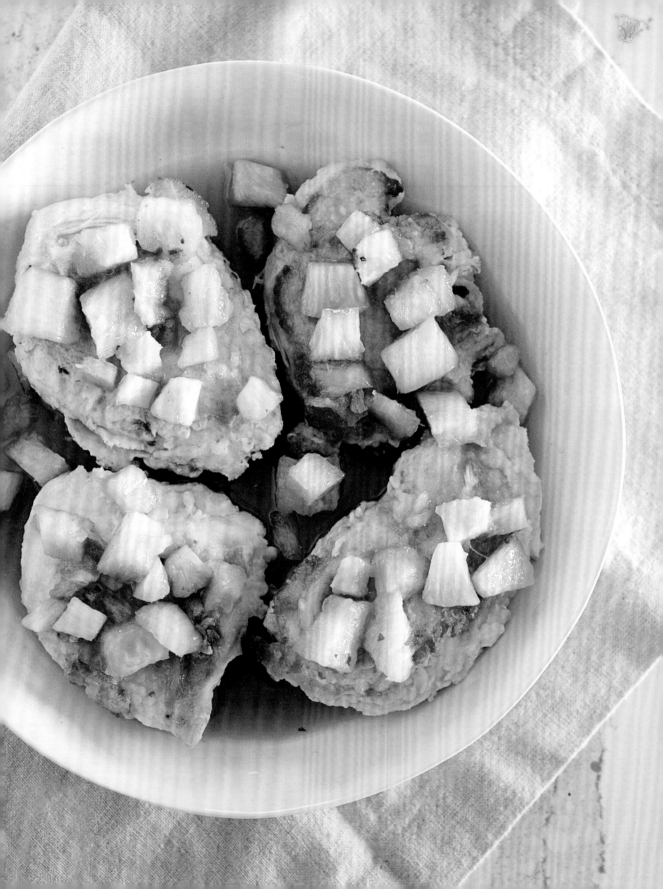

YUMMY PINEAPPLE CHICKEN

Your family will love this recipe for naturally sweet, super-yummy, fresh pineapple chicken. This chicken goes perfectly over steamed rice or quinoa. FODMAP fact: Pineapple is low-FODMAP, at 1 cup (140 g) per serving. But opt for fresh pineapple, as canned versions have not been tested.

Place the chicken between two pieces of wax paper or plastic wrap and tenderize with a mallet or meat tenderizer to a uniform thickness. Place the flour in a shallow dish and dredge the chicken in the flour to coat both sides well.

Heat the oil in a large skillet over medium-high heat and fry the chicken pieces until lightly browned on both sides, about 4 minutes per side. Transfer to a covered dish to keep warm. Wipe out the pan.

Meanwhile, in a small bowl, combine the pineapple juice and cornstarch and stir until smooth. Add the juice mixture to the clean pan. Stir in the corn syrup and tamari and bring the mixture to a boil over medium-high heat. Cook and stir until thickened, about 30 seconds. Add the chunks of pineapple and then the cooked chicken pieces. Stir until everything is warmed through. Remove from the heat and serve.

NOTE To test pineapple for ripeness, sniff the "butt end" of the pineapple (the end without the leaves). It should smell sweet and fragrant when ripe.

TIP To juice fresh pineapple, I recommend cubing the pineapple, then blending or mashing it. Place in a fine strainer over a bowl and press the pulp with the back of a spoon to obtain the juice. Easy!

Four 4-ounce (112 g) boneless skinless chicken breasts

1 tablespoon (8 g) all-purpose gluten-free low-FODMAP flour

2 tablespoons (30 ml) canola oil

¼ cup (60 ml) juice from pineapple (1 cup [140 g] of fresh pineapple will yield this amount of juice; see Note)

1 teaspoon cornstarch

1 tablespoon (15 ml) light corn syrup

1 tablespoon (15 ml) tamari (gluten-free soy sauce) or soy sauce

2 cups (280 g) chopped fresh pineapple

VARIATION

+ For a little kick, chop a medium red bell pepper and add it to the pan just before the pineapple chunks. Let this simmer for 2 to 3 minutes to soften the pepper, then continue with the recipe.

CRISPY CHICKEN NUGGETS

Everyone's favorite meal, these chicken nuggets are crispy and delicious. I pair them with my Microwave Sweet and Sour Sauce (page 163), but they also go great with my Copycat Secret Sauce (page 169) and Bold BBQ Sauce (page 163).

Six 4-ounce (112 g) boneless skinless chicken breasts, cut into 1-inch (2.5 cm) cubes

1 teaspoon salt

2 eggs

1 cup (128 g) cornstarch

Canola oil, for frying

¾ cup (180 ml) Microwave Sweet and Sour Sauce (page 163), for dipping

Sprinkle the chicken with the salt. Crack the eggs into a shallow bowl and whisk well. Place the cornstarch in a second shallow bowl. Piece by piece, dip the chicken in the eggs, then the cornstarch, coating well. Set the coated chicken pieces on wax paper or a cutting board.

Place a skillet over medium-high heat and add oil to a depth of ½ inch (1.3 cm). Place the chicken pieces in the oil and fry on all sides until browned, crispy, and fully cooked, 3 to 4 minutes per side. Drain the chicken and blot with paper towels, then serve with the sauce.

NOTE These nuggets go well with my Crispy Baked Garlic French Fries (page 65) on the side.

VARIATION

+ If you prefer to avoid corn products, use potato starch instead of cornstarch.

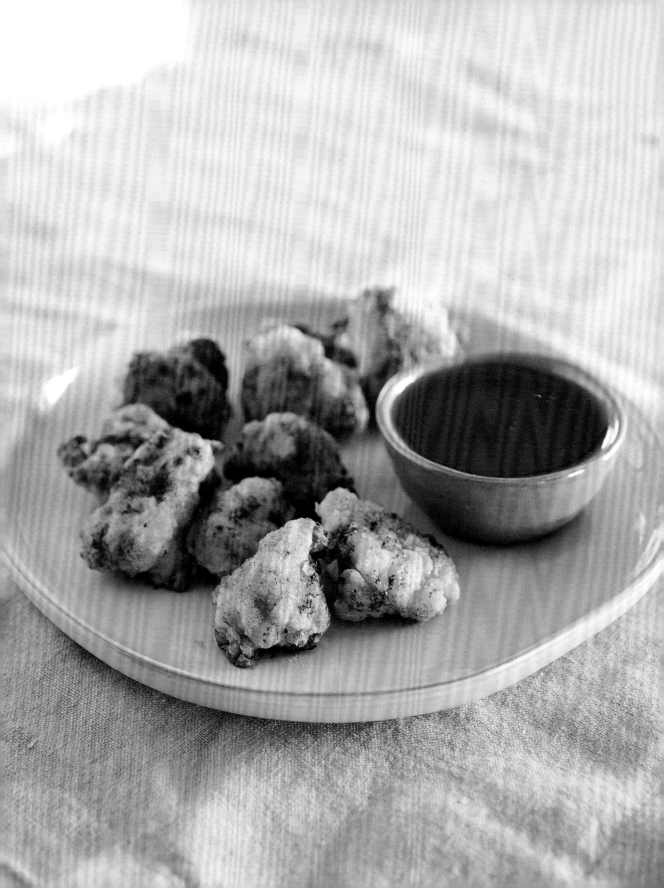

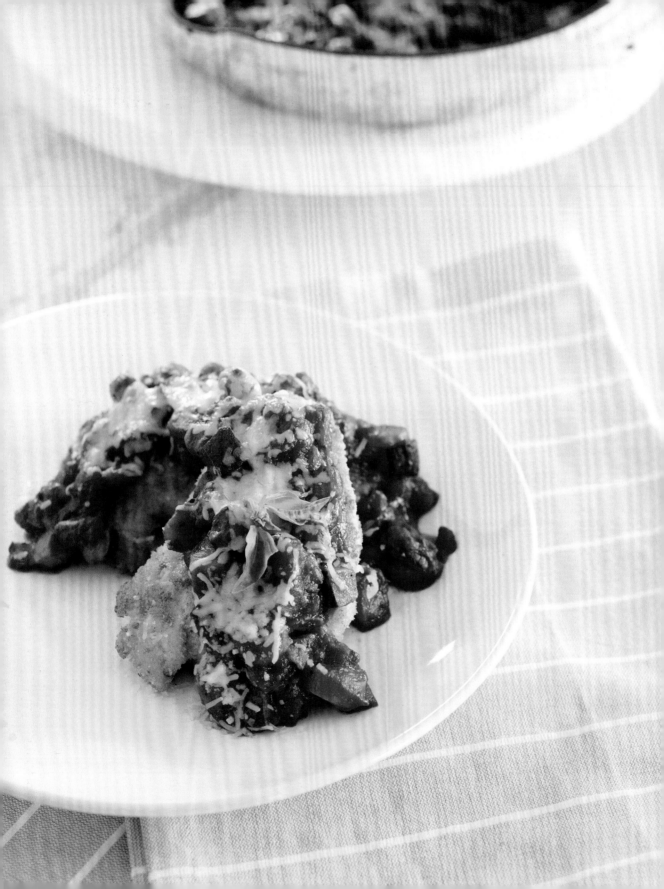

NO-BAKE CHICKEN PARMESAN

Yes, you read that correctly. A chicken Parmesan dinner for the whole family that doesn't require an oven. One pan. Easy cleanup. Delicious. You are going to love this recipe!

Place the chicken between two pieces of wax paper or plastic wrap and tenderize with a mallet or meat tenderizer to a uniform thickness. Place the beaten eggs in one small bowl and the breadcrumbs in a second bowl. Dip the chicken breasts in the egg, then the breadcrumbs, and set aside.

Heat the oil in a large skillet (with a lid) over medium-high heat. Add the chicken pieces and fry until lightly browned on both sides, about 4 minutes per side. Spoon the sauce over the chicken in the skillet, then sprinkle with the cheese. Cover the pan with its lid and turn the heat to medium-low. Cook until the chicken is cooked through and the cheese is melted, about 5 minutes. Serve immediately.

NOTE This is delicious with sautéed spinach on the side or garnished with fresh basil.

TIP If you don't have time to make my Red Wine Marinara, you can substitute a purchased sauce. Just be aware that most marinaras contain high-FODMAP ingredients. Select a low-FODMAP brand (see my shopping guide on page 25).

Six 4-ounce (112 g) boneless skinless chicken breasts or thighs

2 eggs, beaten

½ cup (60 g) gluten-free low-FODMAP breadcrumbs

1 tablespoon (15 ml) olive oil

1½ cups (180 ml) Red Wine Marinara (page 160)

1 cup (120 g) shredded mozzarella

VARIATION

+ For a spicier sauce, add 1 tablespoon (15 ml) hot sauce or 1 teaspoon red pepper flakes.

DELICIOUS MEAT AND POULTRY

THE BEST BURGERS

These are my family's favorite burgers, and we have them almost every week—my husband typically enjoys two or more at one sitting. They are delicious cooked on the stovetop or grill. Use mayonnaise, mustard, or another condiment with these burgers to limit the total amount of ketchup consumed.

FOR THE BURGERS

1 pound (455 g) extra-lean ground beef

1 egg, beaten

3 tablespoons (15 g) traditional (old-fashioned) rolled oats

3 tablespoons (45 ml) ketchup

½ teaspoon salt

¼ teaspoon pepper

1 tablespoon (15 ml) canola oil, for frying (optional)

FOR ASSEMBLY

5 gluten-free low-FODMAP buns

Sliced tomatoes

Shredded lettuce

If cooking on a grill, preheat the grill to medium-high.

To make the burgers: Combine the beef, egg, oats, ketchup, salt, and pepper in a medium bowl and mix well. Form into five patties. If cooking on the stovetop, heat the oil in a large skillet over medium-high heat. Grill or cook to your preferred doneness: for medium-rare, about 3 minutes per side; for medium, about 4 minutes per side; for well done, about 5 minutes per side.

To assemble: Place each burger on a bun and top with tomato and lettuce.

NOTE These are perfect with my Copycat Secret Sauce (page 169).

VARIATIONS

+ If you prefer to avoid beef, try these burgers with ground chicken or turkey instead.

+ Make it a cheeseburger with a slice of your favorite cheese added toward the end of cooking.

ONE-PAN MAPLE MUSTARD CHICKEN

This one-pan meal has just the right amount of sweetness and goes perfectly with steamed rice or potatoes and sautéed spinach. The sauce is so good, you may lick the plate! FODMAP fact: Yellow mustard is low in FODMAPs in servings of 1 tablespoon (11 g); check the ingredient list to ensure there is minimal onion and garlic added to your mustard brand.

In a medium bowl, whisk together the maple syrup, two mustards, and dill. Add more syrup or mustard to taste if necessary; set aside.

Heat the oil in a large skillet over medium-high heat. Add the chicken and cook for 3 to 5 minutes on each side. Season with salt and pepper, then pour in the maple mustard sauce. Stir to ensure the chicken breasts are evenly coated and continue cooking until the chicken is warmed through, 1 minute.

NOTE Chicken is cooked through when the juices run clear. For easier cooking, you can pound the chicken to a uniform thickness prior to frying.

½ cup (120 ml) maple syrup

¼ cup (44 g) yellow mustard

¼ cup (44 g) Dijon mustard

1 teaspoon chopped fresh dill

2 tablespoons (30 ml) canola oil

Four 5- to 6-ounce (140 to 168 g) boneless skinless chicken breasts

Salt and pepper to taste

VARIATIONS

+ Try this with a seeded grainy mustard instead of Dijon.

+ If you don't have fresh dill, you can use ⅓ teaspoon dried dill instead.

DELICIOUS MEAT AND POULTRY

ASIAN BEEF WITH NOODLES

Tasty beef with vegetables and noodles in a savory sauce makes a perfect weeknight meal. It is super easy, filling, *and* delicious. FODMAP fact: Oyster sauce is low-FODMAP in 1-tablespoon (15 ml) servings.

FOR THE SAUCE

3 tablespoons (45 ml) tamari (gluten-free soy sauce)
or soy sauce

1 tablespoon (15 ml) oyster sauce (gluten-free if necessary)

1 tablespoon (15 g) packed brown sugar

1 teaspoon freshly grated ginger

1 teaspoon toasted sesame oil

FOR THE BEEF AND NOODLES

8 ounces (224 g) low-FODMAP Asian rice noodles or gluten-free spaghetti

2 tablespoons (30 ml) garlic-infused olive oil (page 25), divided

1 pound (455 g) beef top sirloin fillet, thinly sliced across the grain

1 cup (75 g) broccoli florets

2 medium carrots, peeled and diced

Salt and pepper to taste

To make the sauce: Whisk together the tamari, oyster sauce, brown sugar, ginger, and sesame oil in a small bowl and set aside.

To make the beef and noodles: Cook the noodles per package directions, drain, and toss with 1 tablespoon (15 ml) of the infused oil. Heat the remaining 1 tablespoon (15 ml) infused oil in a large skillet over medium-high heat. Add the beef and cook until browned, 3 to 4 minutes, flipping as needed. Transfer the beef to a covered dish and set aside.

Add the broccoli and carrots to the skillet. Cook, stirring frequently, until tender, 3 to 4 minutes. Return the beef to the skillet and add the noodles. Stir in the sauce and cook for 2 to 3 minutes, until the meat, noodles, and vegetables are well coated with the sauce.

NOTE I prefer low-sodium soy sauce for my recipes.

VARIATIONS

+ Try this with chicken instead of beef if you prefer to avoid red meat.

+ Select zucchini instead of broccoli for a different flavor.

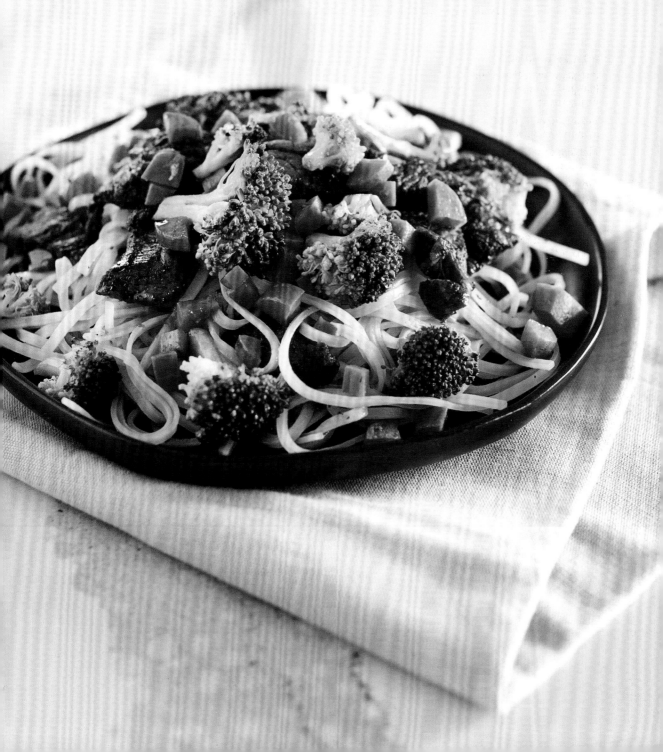

HEARTY BEEF, QUINOA, AND LENTIL CASSEROLE

This is a tasty, hearty, and satisfying casserole that incorporates a trio of protein and energy sources: ground beef, quinoa, *and* lentils. It's a powerhouse! You will love serving this to your family. It also freezes well.

½ cup (86 g) raw quinoa

1½ cups (360 ml) low-FODMAP beef or chicken stock, homemade (page 167) or store-bought (page 21)

2 tablespoons (30 ml) garlic-infused olive oil (page 25), divided

12 ounces (340 g) lean ground beef

⅓ cup (13 g) torn or chopped fresh basil

2 teaspoons (4 g) low-FODMAP Italian seasoning, homemade (page 49) or store-bought

Salt and pepper to taste

1 medium red bell pepper, cored and diced

1 carrot, peeled and diced

¾ cup (138 g) canned lentils, rinsed and drained

6 tablespoons (90 g) tomato paste

¾ cup (180 ml) water

¼ cup (60 ml) red wine

Place the quinoa in a medium saucepan with the stock and bring to a boil, then lower the heat to a simmer and cook until the quinoa is tender, 15 to 20 minutes.

Meanwhile, in a large skillet, heat 1 tablespoon (15 ml) of the infused oil and then add the ground beef. Cover with a lid and cook over medium heat until no longer pink, 7 to 10 minutes. Remove the lid and add the remaining 1 tablespoon (15 ml) infused oil, basil, Italian seasoning, and a few pinches of salt. Continue to cook, stirring, for 2 to 3 more minutes. Mix in the bell pepper and carrot, then add the lentils and mix it all together.

In a small bowl, stir together the tomato paste and water, then add to the skillet and continue to simmer for 3 to 4 more minutes. Add the wine, then taste the sauce and add salt and pepper as needed. Simmer for about 5 minutes, then add the cooked quinoa and fold it all together. Serve hot.

VARIATION

+ Top each portion with ¼ cup (30 g) shredded mozzarella or Cheddar cheese for a non-dairy-free version.

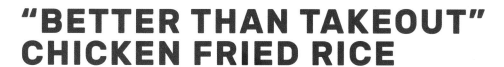

"BETTER THAN TAKEOUT" CHICKEN FRIED RICE

Chicken fried rice is a one-pan meal you will love to make. Not only is it simple, but the taste is delicious. Rice, veggies, and chicken come together to create a healthy and satisfying meal that will please your whole family. It's better than your favorite takeout!

In a large nonstick wok or skillet, heat 2 teaspoons (10 ml) of the sesame oil and 2 teaspoons (10 ml) of the infused oil over medium-high heat. Add the chicken and season lightly with salt and pepper. Lower the heat to medium and sauté until cooked through, 5 to 6 minutes. Transfer the chicken to a plate and set aside.

Return the skillet to medium-high heat and add the remaining 3 teaspoons (15 ml) sesame oil and remaining 1 teaspoon (5 ml) infused oil. Add the carrots and sauté for 3 minutes, then add the zucchini and cook until soft, 3 to 4 minutes. Add the corn and chives and sauté for 1 minute longer. Push the veggies to one side of the pan and pour the eggs onto the other side. Lightly season the eggs with salt and pepper and scramble them. Return the chicken to the skillet along with the cooked rice. Add the tamari and stir-fry until everything is warmed and coated with the sauce. Serve immediately.

5 teaspoons (25 ml) toasted sesame oil, divided

1 tablespoon (15 ml) garlic-infused olive oil (page 25), divided

1 pound (455 g) boneless skinless chicken breasts, chopped into pieces

Salt and pepper to taste

1 cup (120 g) chopped carrot (2 to 3 medium)

1 medium zucchini, chopped

½ cup (64 g) fresh or fresh frozen corn kernels

2 tablespoons (8 g) chopped chives or green scallion tips

2 eggs, whisked

4 cups (660 g) cooked rice of your choice (long-grain, white, or basmati works well)

¼ cup (60 ml) low-sodium tamari (gluten-free soy sauce) or soy sauce

DELICIOUS MEAT AND POULTRY

VARIATION

+ This recipe works well with shrimp or beef strips instead of chicken.

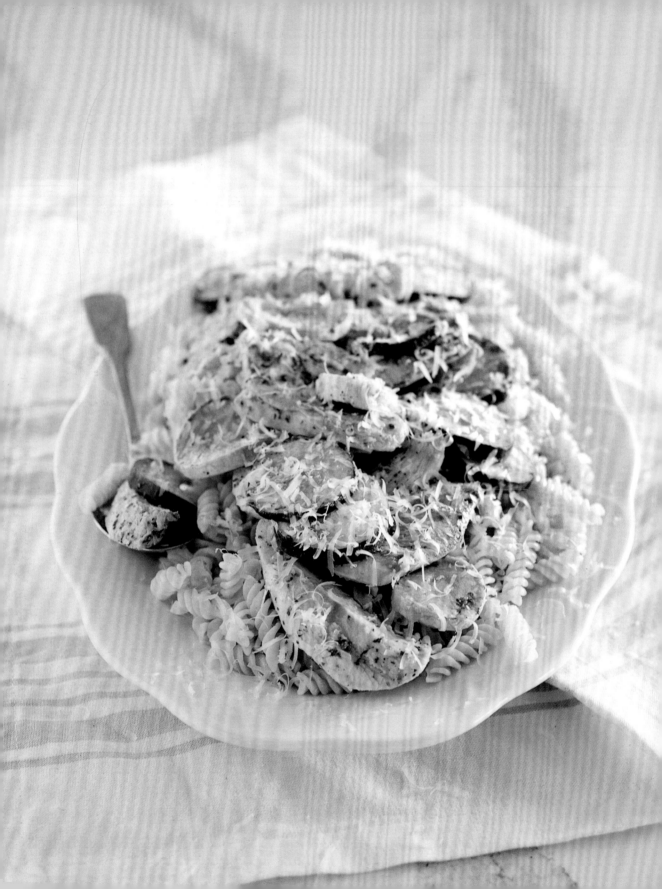

LEMON CHICKEN WITH ROTINI AND VEGETABLES

A gourmet meal, ready in a snap. Everyone loves chicken, pasta, and vegetables enrobed in a rich, creamy, and lemony sauce. FODMAP fact: Yellow squash contains trace FODMAPs and can be eaten freely; however, zucchini is limited to servings of ⅓ cup (65 g) due to levels of fructans.

Bring a large pot of salted water to a boil over high heat. Add the pasta and cook according to package directions, until al dente. Drain and toss with 1 tablespoon (14 g) of the butter to lubricate the pasta. Meanwhile, place the chicken in a large resealable bag with the Italian seasoning, lemon zest, salt, and pepper and massage through the bag to coat the chicken on all sides. Heat 1 tablespoon (15 ml) of the infused oil and the remaining 1 tablespoon (14 g) butter in a large skillet over medium-high heat. Add the seasoned chicken and cook until golden brown, 2 to 3 minutes, then flip and cook the second side, 2 to 3 minutes longer. Transfer the chicken to a covered dish and set aside. Wipe out the pan.

Heat the remaining 1 tablespoon (15 ml) infused oil in the clean pan. Add the zucchini and yellow squash, season with salt and pepper, and drizzle with the lemon juice. Cook until tender, about 3 minutes. Transfer the pasta to a serving platter, cover with the chicken, then the vegetables, and sprinkle with the Parmesan cheese. Serve immediately.

1 pound (455 g) gluten-free low-FODMAP rotini pasta

2 tablespoons (28 g) unsalted butter, divided

1½ pounds (680 g) boneless skinless chicken breasts, cut into strips

1 teaspoon low-FODMAP Italian seasoning, homemade (page 49) or store-bought

1 teaspoon lemon zest (1 lemon is enough for the juice and zest of this recipe)

Salt and pepper to taste

2 tablespoons (30 ml) garlic-infused olive oil (page 25), divided

2 small zucchini, sliced (1⅓ cups [150 g])

2 small yellow squash, sliced

2 tablespoons (30 ml) freshly squeezed lemon juice (about ½ medium lemon)

1 cup (100 g) freshly grated Parmesan cheese

VARIATIONS

+ Use another pasta if you prefer; this goes well with gluten-free farfalle, spaghettini, and penne.

+ For a dairy-free version, substitute vegan margarine or additional olive oil for the butter, and skip the Parmesan cheese.

DELICIOUS MEAT AND POULTRY

TEN-MINUTE SPAGHETTI SAUCE

I grew up making this recipe; it comes together so easily, but tastes so good. Adding corn to spaghetti sauce gives a hint of sweetness and great texture (some call this a "Mexican" spaghetti sauce). FODMAP fact: While canned corn is high-FODMAP, you can enjoy ⅓ cup (40 g) of corn off the cob per serving. Make sure to use fresh or fresh frozen corn in your cooking.

1 tablespoon (15 ml) garlic-infused olive oil (page 25)

1 pound (455 g) extra-lean ground beef

2 cups (480 ml) Red Wine Marinara (page 160)

⅔ cup (80 g) corn kernels (fresh or fresh frozen)

Salt and pepper to taste

4 cups (400 g) cooked low-FODMAP, gluten-free pasta of your choice (see Grocery Shopping List on page 24)

Heat the oil in a large skillet over medium-high heat. Add the beef and cook until browned, about 5 minutes. Add the marinara and corn kernels and simmer for 5 minutes. Season with salt and pepper to taste. Serve over prepared pasta.

NOTE Try it over spaghetti squash for a low-carb option.

TIP My Red Wine Marinara (page 160) is a chunky sauce with vegetables already added. If you substitute store-bought low-FODMAP sauce, try adding ½ cup (60 g) chopped green bell pepper, carrots, or zucchini for added flavor.

VARIATION

+ Sprinkle freshly grated Parmesan over the top if you tolerate dairy.

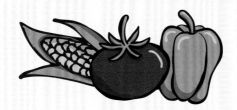

SUPERFOOD VEGAN AND VEGETARIAN MEALS

Following a low-FODMAP diet while vegan or vegetarian may sound impossible at first, but these recipes will show you how delicious life can be! Here are fabulous recipes for your favorite dishes.

QUINOA AND LENTIL KITCHARI

Kitchari is a healing meal according to ancient Indian Ayurveda tradition. It refers to a mixture of two grains. This recipe is so simple but incredibly flavorful. FODMAP fact: Lentils are low-FODMAP in ¼-cup (46 g) servings, provided you use the canned variety. The FODMAPs will leach from the lentils during canning and be removed when you drain the liquid. Do not substitute dried lentils, as their allocated portion size is much smaller.

1 cup (165 g) raw quinoa

2 cups (480 ml) low-FODMAP vegan stock

1 carrot, peeled and diced

½ red bell pepper, chopped

2 tablespoons (30 ml) garlic-infused olive oil (page 25)

¼ cup (15 g) minced fresh parsley

1 cup (184 g) canned lentils, drained and rinsed

Salt and pepper to taste

Place the quinoa, stock, carrot, and red pepper in a medium pot over medium-high heat. Cook the quinoa for 25 minutes, until the liquid is absorbed. The mixture should be slightly thin; add more stock if needed to achieve that consistency. Stir in the infused oil, parsley, lentils, and salt and pepper and warm over low heat for 2 to 3 minutes.

NOTE Serve this with tamari or soy sauce on the side.

VARIATION

+ Add 1 teaspoon turmeric, ½ teaspoon ground cumin, and 1 teaspoon garam masala for a different flavor.

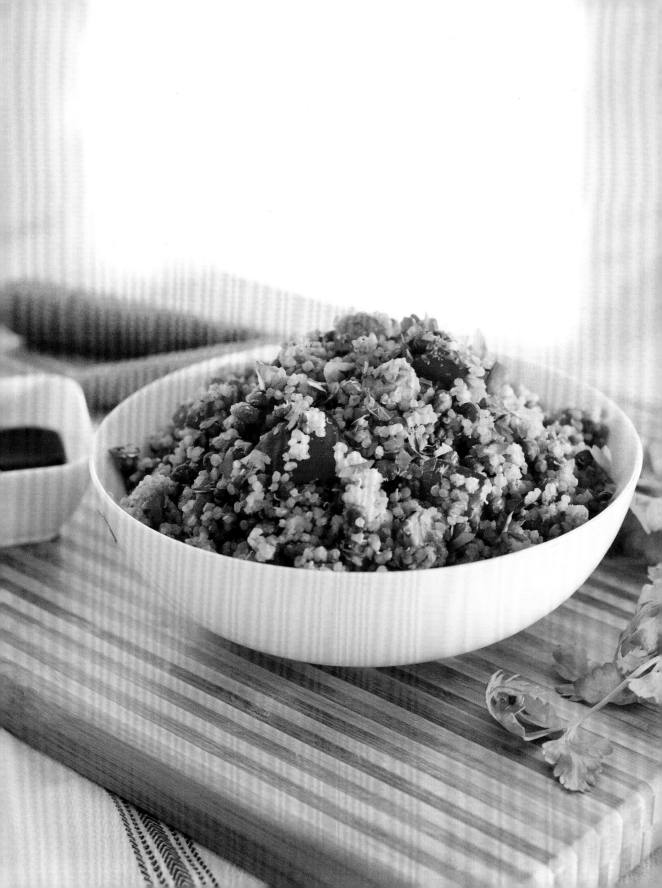

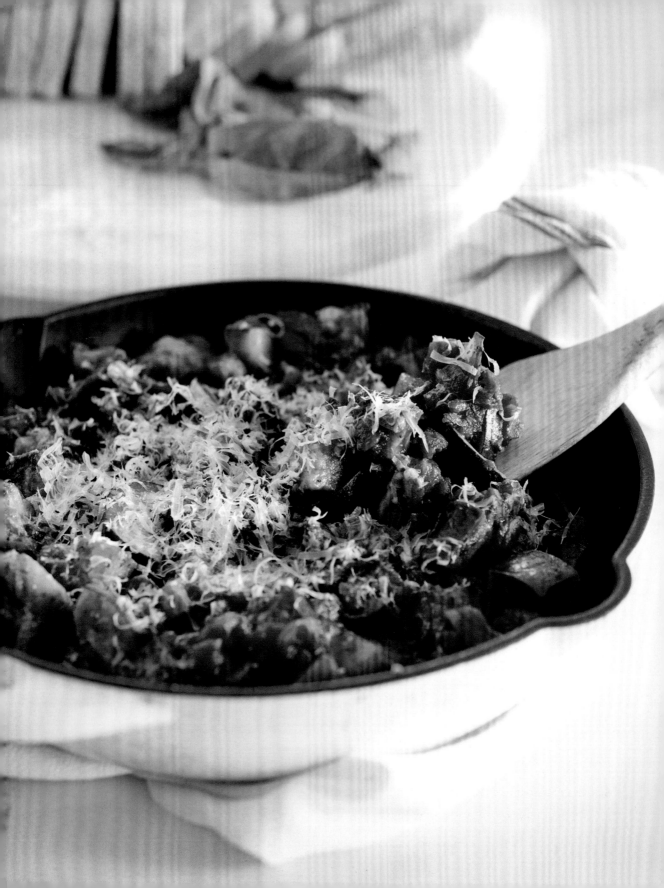

ONE-POT RATATOUILLE

This recipe combines the wonderful flavors of tomato, eggplant, and zucchini, with the richness of cheese. It will be one of your favorites. FODMAP fact: Up to 1 cup (75 g) of cooked cubed eggplant is low-FODMAP, due to sorbitol levels. Zucchini is limited to ⅓-cup (65 g) servings, due to higher amounts of fructans. Even though they seem similar, they actually have very different carbohydrates.

Place the eggplant in a strainer/colander and sprinkle with 1 teaspoon (6 g) of the salt. Let stand for 5 minutes, then press out any excess liquid using your hands and a paper towel.

Heat the oil in a large Dutch oven or skillet over medium heat. Add the zucchini, eggplant, basil, and Italian seasoning. Season with the remaining 1½ teaspoons (9 g) salt and the pepper. Cook until the vegetables are tender, stirring occasionally, about 10 minutes. Add the wine. Cook, stirring often, until the wine is absorbed, about 2 minutes. Add the canned tomatoes and let the sauce simmer over low heat for another 5 minutes. Taste the sauce, and add more Italian seasoning, salt, or pepper as desired. Remove from the heat, sprinkle with the cheeses, and let stand until the cheese melts.

NOTES

+ This is wonderful with low-FODMAP bread, such as gluten-free rolls or white sourdough (read about sourdough and FODMAPs on page 126).

+ If the cheese isn't melting, pop the uncovered Dutch oven under the broiler for 1 to 2 minutes.

1 medium eggplant, chopped into bite-size pieces (4 cups [300 g])

2½ teaspoons (15 g) salt, divided, plus more to taste

2 tablespoons (30 ml) garlic-infused olive oil (page 25)

1 medium zucchini, halved and seeds scraped out

3 or 4 leaves fresh basil, chopped

2 tablespoons (8 g) low-FODMAP Italian seasoning, homemade (page 49) or store-bought, plus more to taste

1 teaspoon freshly ground black pepper, plus more to taste

½ cup (120 ml) red wine

One 14.5-ounce (406 g) can diced tomatoes (no added onion, garlic)

1½ cups (180 g) shredded Swiss cheese

¼ cup (25 g) grated Parmesan cheese

VARIATIONS

+ Skip the cheese for a fully vegan version.

+ Instead of the Swiss cheese, try mozzarella.

POLENTA MARINARA BOWL

Polenta is an Italian dish consisting of boiled cornmeal. It is creamy and delicious, plus packed with protein, fiber, and vitamins. FODMAP fact: One cup (255 g) of cooked polenta is one low-FODMAP serving.

3 cups (720 ml) water

1 cup (140 g) polenta corn grits

½ teaspoon salt

1 tablespoon (15 ml) olive oil

2 tablespoons (2 g) nutritional yeast

2 cups (480 ml) Red Wine Marinara (page 160)

¼ cup (25 g) chopped black olives

½ cup (20 g) chopped fresh basil

Add the water to a medium pot and bring to a boil over medium-high heat. Add the polenta and salt, whisking well to ensure no clumping. Decrease the heat to medium-low and cook for about 20 minutes, whisking frequently. Once the polenta has thickened, stir in the olive oil and nutritional yeast and set aside.

Warm the marinara sauce in the microwave or a second small pot. Divide the polenta among four bowls, pour the marinara on top, and sprinkle with the olives and basil.

VARIATION

+ Add 1⅓ cups (160 g) shredded mozzarella cheese for a vegetarian version.

BBQ TOFU "STEAKS"

These BBQ tofu steaks go great in a burger bun, layered with lettuce, alfalfa sprouts, and mayonnaise. FODMAP fact: Commercially available barbecue sauce is low-FODMAP in servings of 2 tablespoons (30 ml).

Cooking spray

One 14-ounce (392 g) package extra-firm tofu, drained

½ cup (120 ml) Bold BBQ Sauce (page 163)

1 tablespoon (2 g) nutritional yeast

Preheat the oven or toaster oven to 400°F (200°C or gas mark 6). Line a baking sheet with foil and spray the foil with cooking spray.

Slice the tofu into four rectangles or strips about 1 inch (2.5 cm) thick. Combine the barbecue sauce and nutritional yeast in a small bowl, and brush on both sides of each tofu piece. Lay the tofu strips on the baking sheet and bake for 20 to 25 minutes, until crisp.

VARIATION

+ Try this with my Copycat Secret Sauce (page 169) instead of mayonnaise on your bun.

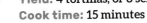
CHEESE AND SPINACH QUESADILLAS

Quesadillas are an ideal dinner choice that will please your whole family. Adding spinach gives this recipe delicious flavor *and* nutritional punch. I love that corn tortillas are readily available, so these will be naturally low-FODMAP and gluten-free.

Heat the oil in a medium nonstick skillet over medium heat. Add the spinach and cook until wilted, about 5 minutes. Transfer the spinach to a covered plate and set aside.

Place one tortilla on the pan and spread ½ cup (30 g) of the cheese on the tortilla, then add one-fourth of the spinach and one-fourth of the tomatoes. Lay a second tortilla over the first and press down with a spatula. Cover the skillet with a lid and cook until the cheese melts and the bottom of the tortilla is browned, about 3 minutes. Flip gently and cook the other side for about 3 minutes. Transfer to a covered plate and repeat with the remaining ingredients. Cut into quarters to serve.

NOTE Serve these with my Restaurant-Style Salsa (page 160).

1 tablespoon (15 ml) olive oil

8 ounces (224 g) fresh baby spinach, rinsed and dried

Eight 8-inch (20 cm) soft corn tortillas or gluten-free low-FODMAP flour tortillas

2 cups (240 g) shredded Cheddar cheese

1 medium tomato, chopped

SUPERFOOD VEGAN AND VEGETARIAN MEALS

VARIATION

+ Skip the spinach and add green scallion tips or minced red pepper instead.

CHICKPEA AND QUINOA CURRY

This chickpea and quinoa curry is absolutely fantastic. The flavors are rich and complex, yet the recipe is so easy. Only one pot required! FODMAP fact: I love using canned tomatoes in cooking; you can enjoy ⅗ cup (about 4 ounces [115 g]) per serving.

2 tablespoons (30 ml) garlic-infused olive oil (page 25)

1 cup (120 g) peeled and chopped carrot (about 2 large carrots)

1 tablespoon (6 g) peeled and minced fresh ginger

2 teaspoons (4 g) yellow curry powder

1 teaspoon ground cumin

3 cups (720 ml) low-FODMAP vegan stock

1 cup (173 g) uncooked quinoa

One 28-ounce (784 g) can diced tomatoes (no added spices)

12 ounces (250 g) canned chickpeas, drained and rinsed

½ cup (120 ml) canned coconut milk

Salt and pepper to taste

Heat the oil in a large saucepan or Dutch oven over medium heat. Add the carrot and ginger and cook for 5 to 10 minutes, until starting to soften. Stir in the curry powder and cumin and let sit for 1 to 2 minutes. Add the stock, quinoa, and diced tomatoes and lightly simmer for 15 minutes, until the quinoa is tender. Stir in the chickpeas and coconut milk and warm for 1 to 2 minutes. Season with salt and pepper to taste.

NOTE Serve this curry immediately, or keep it in the refrigerator for 5 days or freezer for 3 months.

VARIATION

+ Try this recipe with brown rice instead of quinoa, or use a combination!

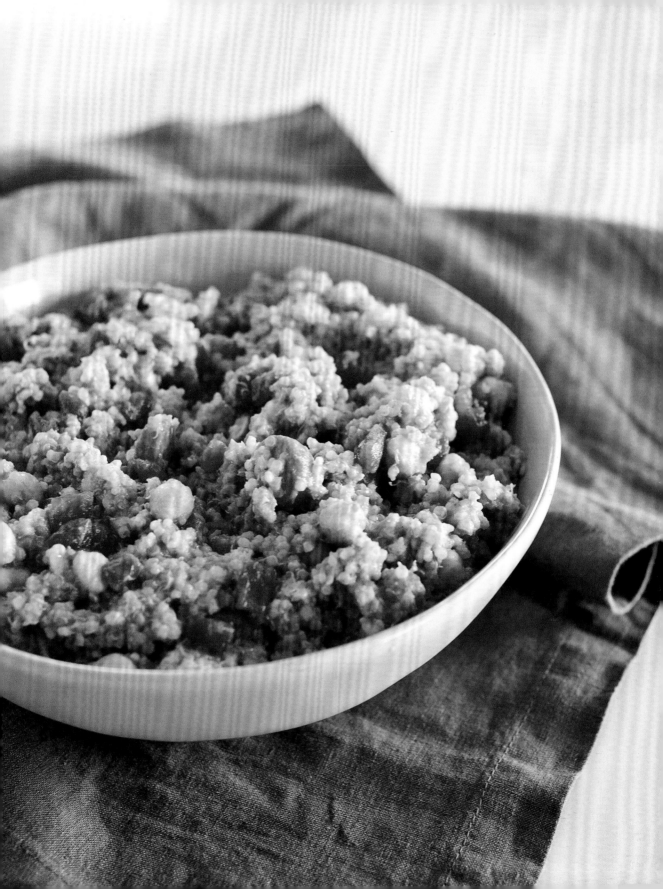

HERBY RICOTTA AND VEGETABLE HOAGIE

Sometimes the simple things are what you want. This recipe incorporates my versatile vegan ricotta, made with fresh herbs and tofu (page 162). I love to layer this ricotta on fresh crusty bread with assorted vegetables. FODMAP fact: White wheat sourdough bread is low-FODMAP if the bread is proofed for about 12 hours (check with your bakery). The fermentation process of "souring" the dough reduces the fructans in the wheat and therefore makes it lower in FODMAPs. It still would contain gluten, so avoid if you are gluten-sensitive.

One 6-inch (15 cm) sourdough baguette, cut in half (if not avoiding gluten) or gluten-free low-FODMAP bagel

2 tablespoons (30 g) Herby Tofu Vegan Ricotta (page 162)

½ cup (15 g) butter lettuce

2 or 3 slices ripe tomato

⅛ cucumber, sliced

2 tablespoons (8 g) alfalfa sprouts

Olive oil, for drizzling

Salt and pepper to taste

Place the bread on a plate. Spread one side with ricotta. Top with the lettuce, tomatoes, cucumber, and sprouts. Drizzle with oil and season with salt and pepper. Put the halves together, and enjoy.

VARIATIONS

+ Make it a wrap instead with a low-FODMAP flatbread or tortilla.

+ Try this hoagie with grilled zucchini, bell peppers, and eggplant instead.

PESTO PENNE WITH TOFU

I am so happy we can buy gluten-free low-FODMAP penne pasta. Combining penne with the flavors of this pesto is delicious and so healthy. I added some tofu to provide texture and extra protein. This meal is simple yet elegant.

Bring a large pot of salted water to a boil over high heat. Add the penne and cook according to the package directions until al dente (do not overcook). Drain, stir in ½ teaspoon of the oil, and set aside.

Heat the remaining 1 teaspoon oil in a medium saucepan over medium-high heat. Add the tamari and tofu and cook until the tofu is browned on all sides, turning as needed, about 20 minutes.

Pour the pesto sauce over the penne and stir until combined. Add the tofu and stir again. Serve immediately, or refrigerate.

NOTE Once cooled, this can be refrigerated in individual serving containers for packed weekday lunches.

12 ounces (340 g) gluten-free low-FODMAP penne

1½ teaspoons garlic-infused olive oil (page 25), divided

1 tablespoon (15 ml) tamari (gluten-free soy sauce) or soy sauce

One 14-ounce (392 g) package extra-firm tofu, drained and cut into cubes

1½ cups (360 g) Kale and Basil Pesto with Walnuts (page 166)

SUPERFOOD VEGAN AND VEGETARIAN MEALS

VARIATIONS

+ Try this with Red Wine Marinara (page 160) instead of pesto.

+ Garnish with fresh basil and toasted pine nuts.

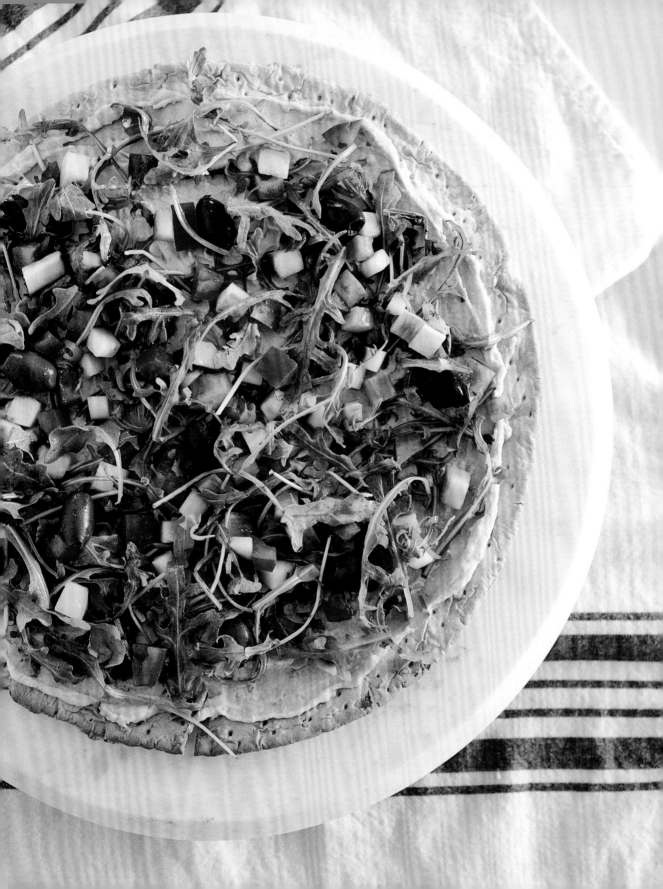

HUMMUS PIZZA WITH GREEK SALAD

Here's a fun, healthy, and delicious way to enjoy hummus dip—as a salad "pizza." This comes together in just 15 minutes, and is great for lunch or a light supper. Some days I whip up the Greek salad to enjoy simply on its own!

Preheat the oven to 400°F (200°C or gas mark 6), or according to the directions of your pizza crust.

Brush the pizza crust with 1 tablespoon (15 ml) of the olive oil and bake until crisp, about 5 minutes (depending on your pizza crust choice). Spread the crust with the hummus.

In a medium bowl, toss together the cucumber, tomato, olives, and arugula; dress with the remaining 1 tablespoon (15 ml) olive oil, the infused oil, and the lemon juice. Season with salt and pepper to taste. Top the hummus with the salad, then sprinkle on the feta and serve immediately.

NOTE Store-bought hummus is not low-FODMAP, so make sure you use the recipe on 159 to keep your tummy happy.

TIP Make this vegan by skipping the feta and selecting a pizza crust or low-FODMAP flatbread made without eggs.

One 9-inch (23 cm) gluten-free low-FODMAP thin pizza crust

2 tablespoons (30 ml) olive oil, divided

¼ cup (60 g) "Humm in Your Head" Hummus (page 159)

½ cup (60 g) chopped cucumber

½ tomato, chopped

¼ cup (25 g) kalamata olives

1 cup (30 g) baby arugula

1 tablespoon (15 ml) garlic-infused olive oil (page 25)

2 tablespoons (30 ml) freshly squeezed lemon juice (about ½ medium lemon)

Salt and pepper to taste

¼ cup (38 g) crumbled feta cheese

SUPERFOOD VEGAN AND VEGETARIAN MEALS

PEANUT PAD THAI

Pad Thai is one of my favorite meals, so this recipe was one of the very first I modified to be low-FODMAP. The peanut sauce is rich and creamy, and it is perfect with additional chopped peanuts on top. FODMAP fact: Bean sprouts contain only trace amounts of FODMAPs, so you can enjoy as much as you wish.

6 ounces (168 g) brown rice noodles

1 teaspoon garlic-infused olive oil (page 25)

12 ounces (340 g) extra-firm tofu, drained and cut into cubes

1 egg, beaten

¾ cup (180 ml) Asian Peanut Dressing (page 162)

½ cup (25 g) bean sprouts

Chopped peanuts, for garnish (optional)

Chopped fresh cilantro, for garnish (optional)

Bring a medium pot of water to a boil and cook the rice noodles until al dente according to package instructions. Drain and leave in the pot.

Meanwhile, heat the oil in a large nonstick skillet over medium-high heat. Add the tofu and cook, turning once, until both sides are brown, about 5 minutes. Slide the tofu to one side of the pan and place the beaten egg on the other side. Scramble the egg lightly. Add the drained noodles to the skillet and pour the dressing over the noodles. Cook for 3 to 5 minutes, until the sauce thickens slightly. Remove from the heat and stir in the bean sprouts. Sprinkle with peanuts and cilantro, if desired.

TIP For a vegan version, skip the egg.

VARIATION

+ Try it with Crispy Sweet and Sour Tofu Nuggets (page 133) instead!

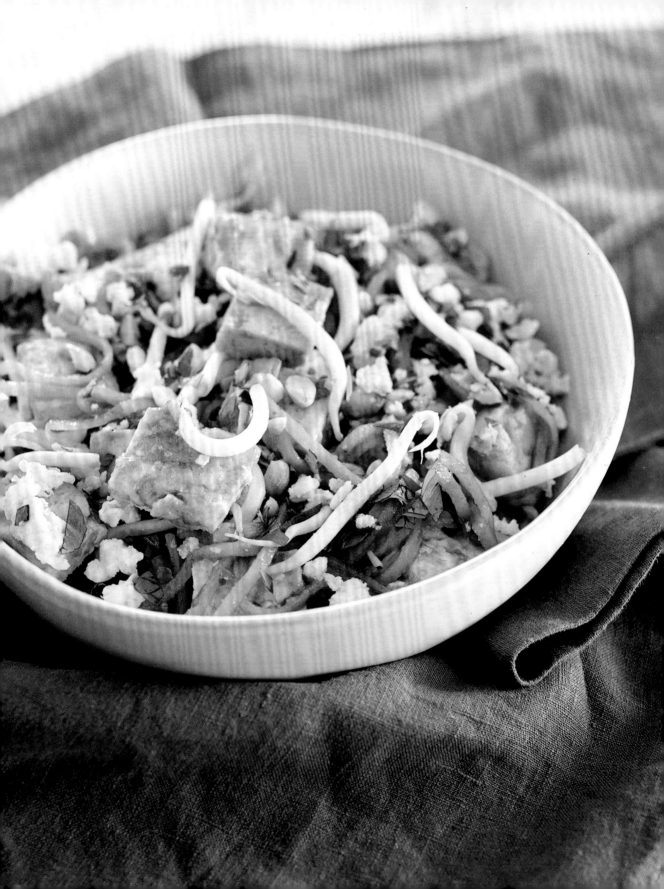

SESAME GINGER TEMPEH STIR-FRY

This is a delicious and easy stir-fry that uses tempeh to provide texture and protein. Tempeh is made with fermented soybeans and has a strong and nutty flavor. It is a bit firmer than tofu and works great as a meat substitute for vegan recipes. FODMAP fact: Four ounces (112 g) of tempeh is one low-FODMAP serving; the fermentation process removes the FODMAPs commonly found in whole soybean products.

2 tablespoons (30 ml) olive oil, divided

8 ounces (224 g) tempeh, cut into bite-size pieces

½ cup (120 ml) Sesame Ginger Dressing or Marinade (page 164), divided

4 cups (480 g) thinly sliced carrots

1½ cups (115 g) broccoli florets

5½ ounces (150 g) green beans (about 30)

In a large skillet, heat 1 tablespoon (15 ml) of the olive oil over medium heat. Add the tempeh and cook for 5 to 10 minutes, flipping to ensure both sides are browned. Spoon 2 tablespoons (30 ml) of the dressing into the pan and cook until the tempeh is coated and the sauce is slightly caramelized, about 5 minutes. Transfer the tempeh to a covered dish and set aside.

Heat the remaining 1 tablespoon (15 ml) olive oil in the skillet and add the carrots, broccoli, and green beans. Add water if needed to help cook the vegetables. Cook for about 5 minutes, then drain any excess water. Return the tempeh to the pan and add the remaining 6 tablespoons (90 ml) sauce. Continue to cook, stirring, until the sauce thickens, about 5 minutes.

NOTE This stir-fry goes perfectly over steamed rice.

TIP Some brands of tempeh contain added garlic or onion seasonings. Be careful to select a tempeh without them.

CRISPY SWEET AND SOUR TOFU NUGGETS

You will make this recipe again and again. Crispy tofu nuggets are a wonderful stand-alone dinner, or a great addition to other dishes. I enjoy this tofu with my Asian Vegetable Stir-Fry (page 66), Peanut Pad Thai (page 130), or steamed rice. FODMAP fact: Extra-firm or firm tofu is low-FODMAP in ⅔-cup (160 g) servings. The soaking process for making firm tofu leaches out the FODMAPs. Note that silken tofu is considered high-FODMAP; do not substitute.

Drain the tofu well, blot with paper towels, and cut into bite-size cubes. Combine the cornstarch, flour, sesame seeds, and salt in a medium bowl. Roll the tofu cubes in the cornstarch mixture until coated well.

In a large saucepan, add the oil to a depth of 1 inch (2.5 cm) and heat over medium-high heat. Add the tofu to the hot oil and cook for 1 to 2 minutes per side, turning as needed (do not burn). Place the cooked tofu on paper towels and blot off excess oil. Serve over steamed rice with the sweet and sour sauce, garnished with additional sesame seeds.

NOTE Be careful when cooking with hot oil. I always use oven gloves to protect my hands and a splatter guard over the pan to prevent oil burns.

One 14-ounce (392 g) package extra-firm tofu

¼ cup (32 g) cornstarch

¼ cup (32 g) all-purpose gluten-free low-FODMAP flour

3 tablespoons (24 g) sesame seeds, plus more for garnish

½ teaspoon salt

Up to 1 cup (240 ml) canola oil, for frying (depending on the size of your skillet)

½ cup (120 ml) Microwave Sweet and Sour Sauce (page 163), for dipping

VARIATION

+ This tofu is amazing with my Asian Peanut Dressing (page 162) and Sesame Ginger Dressing or Marinade (page 164) in place of the sweet and sour sauce.

SUPERFOOD VEGAN AND VEGETARIAN MEALS

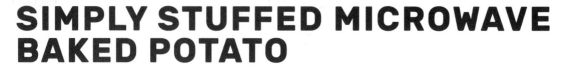
SIMPLY STUFFED MICROWAVE BAKED POTATO

Baked potatoes are a filling, nutritious, and simple meal for both lunch and supper. I love the versatility of a baked potato and the ease of cooking it in the microwave. They are a safe option for eating out as well. FODMAP fact: Sour cream does contain FODMAPs, but you can enjoy up to 2 tablespoons (30 g) in one serving. That is plenty for this baked potato!

One large russet potato (about 14 ounces [392 g])

1 tablespoon (14 g) unsalted butter

1 tablespoon (15 g) sour cream

3 tablespoons (24 g) shredded Cheddar cheese, divided

Salt and pepper to taste

Scrub the potato and prick it several times with a fork. Place it on a microwave-safe plate. Microwave on full power for 11 minutes, or until the potato is soft. Cut the potato lengthwise to within 1 inch (2.5 cm) of the ends (you want to leave the edges of the potato intact to create a pocket to remove the middle). Press lightly on the long ends of the potato to open up the potato along its seam (like a collapsible change purse). Scoop out three-fourths or more of the potato flesh and place in a small bowl. Add the butter, sour cream, and 2 tablespoons (16 g) of the cheese. Mash the potato to your desired texture. Season with salt and pepper. Replace the mashed potato back into the cavity and top with the remaining 1 tablespoon (8 g) cheese. Return it to the microwave, and cook for about 30 seconds to melt the cheese.

NOTE Some potatoes are sold "ready to microwave" wrapped in plastic. If you select one of those potatoes, then you do not need to prick it with a fork.

VARIATION

+ Stir in some steamed broccoli florets and sprinkle with chopped chives.

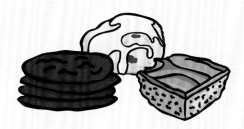

MOUTHWATERING SNACKS AND TREATS

Don't forget to save room for dessert! Just because you are on the low-FODMAP diet does not mean you can't enjoy some delicious snacks and treats. Here are some super-easy and amazing options.

DIY TRAIL MIX

This trail mix is an inexpensive, ready-to-go snack that you can personalize to your preference. I like to use gluten-free pretzels, but if you aren't sensitive to gluten, then you can enjoy ½ cup (24 g) of regular pretzels as a low-FODMAP serving.

1 cup (160 g) salted peanuts

1 cup (160 g) dark chocolate chunks or semisweet chocolate chips

2 cups (2½ to 3 ounces [70 to 84 g] depending on the type of pretzel chosen) gluten-free pretzels

2 cups (54 g) toasted O cereal

½ cup (70 g) dried cranberries

Combine all the ingredients in a large bowl or resealable bag. If desired, portion out into individual bags of single-serving sizes for an easy grab-and-go option.

NOTE Select only salted or unsalted plain peanuts. Honey-roasted peanuts contain honey and fructose, and dry-roasted peanuts contain onion powder.

VARIATIONS

+ Try dark chocolate mini M&M's if you can tolerate small amounts of milk ingredients.

+ Try Corn Chex or another gluten-free cereal instead of toasted O's or pretzels (always check ingredients to ensure the brand of cereal you select does not contain high-FODMAP additives).

PEANUT BUTTER CHOCOLATE CHIP MICROWAVE COOKIE

Imagine a warm, soft, and chewy cookie with the creamy richness of peanut butter and chocolate, ready in 5 minutes, using ingredients you already have. You can do it! Make sure you eat this "cookie" with a spoon, as it will be too soft to pick up (it also tastes delicious with lactose-free ice cream).

Melt the butter in the microwave for about 15 seconds and set aside. Place the egg yolk in a mug or bowl and whisk in both sugars until combined. Add the melted butter, peanut butter, and vanilla and mix again.

In a small bowl, combine the flour, xanthan gum, baking powder, and salt, and then stir the mixture into the wet ingredients. The dough should be slightly thick, like cookie dough. Add the chocolate chips (reserving a few for sprinkling, if desired) and give a final stir. Place the dough in a shallow microwave-safe dish or divide between two ramekins. Cook in the microwave for about 60 seconds. Allow to cool for 3 to 5 minutes before eating.

2 tablespoons (28 g) unsalted butter

1 egg yolk

1 tablespoon (12 g) granulated sugar

1 tablespoon (15 g) brown sugar

2 tablespoons (30 g) all-natural creamy peanut butter (salted or unsalted)

½ teaspoon vanilla extract

2 tablespoons (16 g) gluten-free low-FODMAP flour

⅛ teaspoon xanthan gum (if not added to your flour choice)

¼ teaspoon baking powder

⅛ teaspoon salt (omit if you use salted peanut butter)

2 tablespoons (18 g) semisweet chocolate chips

VARIATIONS

+ If you can't tolerate peanuts, this cookie is also delicious with almond butter or sunflower seed butter.

+ For a dairy-free option, use vegan margarine and dairy-free chocolate chips.

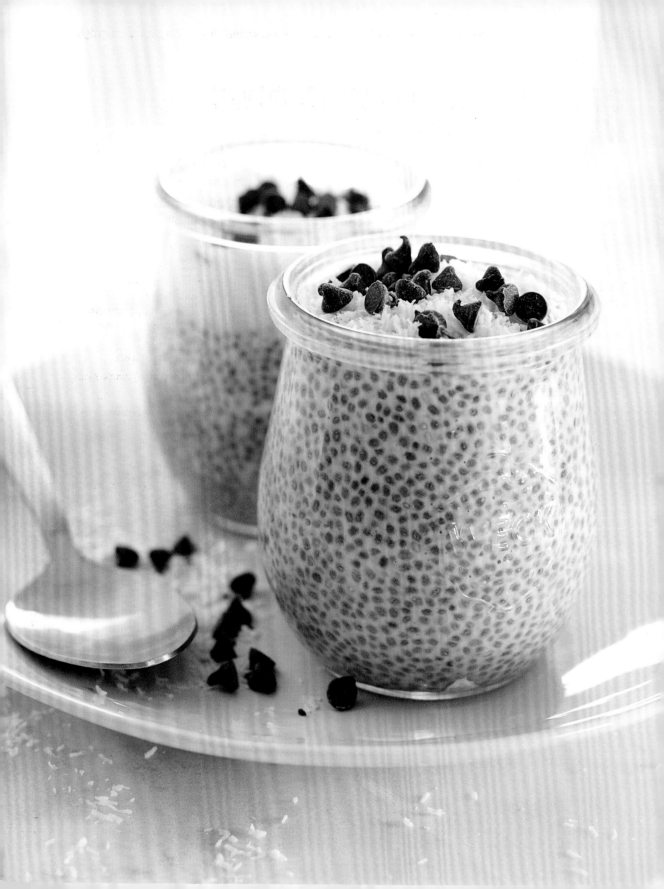

CREAMY CHIA PUDDING WITH COCONUT

Chia seeds are a superfood, known for providing incredible nutrients. One tablespoon (8 g) of chia seeds (only 60 calories) contains 4 grams of fiber, 3 grams of protein, vitamins, essential fatty acids, *and* antioxidants! The seeds absorb liquid like magic, resulting in a soft pudding-like texture. FODMAP fact: Two tablespoons (24 g) are one low-FODMAP serving of chia seeds.

Combine all the ingredients in a bowl or mason jar. Let the mixture sit on the counter for 10 to 15 minutes, giving it a stir every 2 to 3 minutes. This ensures the seeds don't all settle to the bottom and gets them starting to absorb the liquid. Cover and place in the refrigerator until the seeds swell to absorb all the liquid (6 hours or longer). Can keep for 7 days in the refrigerator.

¼ cup (48 g) chia seeds

2 tablespoons (10 g) shredded unsweetened or sweetened coconut

1¼ cups (300 ml) low-FODMAP milk (such as almond milk or lactose-free milk)

1 teaspoon vanilla extract

2 tablespoons (30 ml) maple syrup

VARIATIONS

+ Top the pudding with more shredded coconut, chocolate chips, or fresh raspberries.

+ Skip the coconut for a plain chia seed pudding and use it in one of my smoothie recipes (page 35).

MOUTHWATERING SNACKS AND TREATS

BANANA CHOCOLATE CHIP OAT BARS

These oat bars remind me of banana bread. They are delicious, filling, and packed with healthy energy. Did you know that oat flour contains 21 grams of protein and 12 grams of fiber per cup (120 g)? These are a perfect breakfast, snack, *or* dessert.

Cooking spray

3 very ripe bananas

1 egg (see Tip, page 43, for a vegan egg substitute)

½ cup (115 g) packed brown sugar

3 tablespoons (45 ml) melted unsalted butter or coconut oil (for vegan version)

2 cups (240 g) oat flour (to make your own, see Tip)

1 teaspoon baking powder

½ teaspoon salt

1 teaspoon ground cinnamon

¼ cup (60 ml) low-FODMAP milk (such as almond milk or lactose-free milk)

1 teaspoon vanilla extract

1 cup (150 g) semisweet chocolate chips

Preheat the oven to 350°F (180°C or gas mark 4). Coat a 9 x 13-inch (23 x 33 cm) casserole dish with cooking spray.

Mash the bananas in a small bowl or mug. In a large bowl, whisk together the egg and brown sugar. Add the melted butter, then the mashed bananas and stir. In a separate bowl, combine the oat flour, baking powder, salt, and cinnamon. Add the flour mixture to the wet ingredients and stir to combine. Slowly add the milk and vanilla and stir until well mixed. Fold in the chocolate chips.

Spread the batter in the prepared baking dish and bake for 20 to 25 minutes, or until a toothpick inserted in the center comes out clean (you might get melted chocolate on the toothpick, so disregard that). Let cool for 5 to 10 minutes before slicing and eating.

TIPS

+ *Bonus recipe!* If you don't have oat flour, make your own from traditional rolled oats: Add 2 to 3 cups (160 to 240 g) of traditional oats to a food processor and process at high speed until the oats turn into a fine powder. Store the flour in an airtight container for up to 3 months.

+ *To make ahead:* Cool the bars completely, then wrap each one tightly in plastic wrap. Lay the wrapped bars flat in freezer bags and squeeze out all the air when sealing the bag. Freeze for up to 1 month. When ready to eat, defrost at room temperature (about 1 hour).

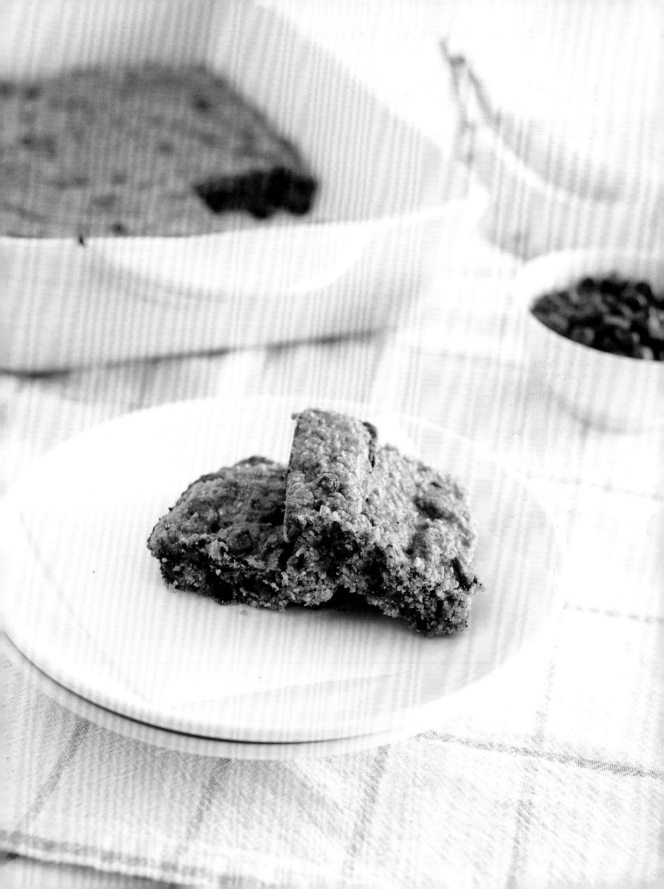

PARMESAN AND GARLIC GOURMET POPCORN

This is a gourmet twist on a favorite snack. I love munching on homemade popcorn because it is healthy *and* filling. Did you know that 3 cups (24 g) of plain popcorn contain 3.6 grams of fiber, 3 grams of protein, and only 100 calories? Up to 7 cups (120 g) is a safe low-FODMAP serving, but due to the added fat of this recipe, limit portions to a smaller amount.

3 tablespoons (45 ml) canola or olive oil

1 teaspoon salt

½ cup (120 g) popcorn kernels

3 tablespoons (42 g) unsalted butter

2 teaspoons (10 ml) garlic-infused olive oil (page 25) or other infused oil (truffle, mushroom)

½ cup (50 g) grated Parmesan cheese

Prepare a bowl on the counter, large enough for the cooked popcorn. Place the canola oil and salt in a large, heavy-bottomed saucepan (3½ quarts [3 L] or larger) with a lid. Set the popcorn kernels next to the stove. Add one popcorn kernel to the oil, and turn the heat to medium-high. When the single kernel pops, the oil is hot and ready. Dump the rest of the kernels into the oil and cover the pot. Shake the pot intermittently to ensure the kernels get cooked evenly and don't burn. When the popping slows down to a few seconds between pops, remove the pot from the heat and dump the popcorn into your large bowl.

In a small glass or bowl, melt the butter and then stir the infused oil into the butter. Toss the butter into the popcorn, then sprinkle the Parmesan cheese on top and mix well. Serve immediately, or let cool completely and place in individual serving bags at room temperature for 2 to 3 days.

NOTE I like to use a pot with a clear lid when making popcorn so that I can see the kernels as they pop.

VARIATION
+ Try this without the Parmesan and infused oil for a classic movie theater–style taste.

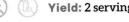
CONFETTI VANILLA MUG CAKE

This is a personal-size confetti vanilla cake that is delicious and fun to eat. Mug cakes are a great option while on the low-FODMAP diet, so you don't feel deprived of your favorite treats. Try it with my simple glaze recipe on page 154.

Crack the egg into a 16-ounce (450 ml) or larger microwave-safe mug, whisk to blend, then measure out 2 tablespoons (30 ml) and discard or reserve the rest for other recipes. Add the sugar to the egg, and whisk to combine well. Add the oil, then mix again. Scoop the flour into your mug, then add the xanthan gum, baking powder, and salt on top of the flour and lightly stir these into the flour, then mix the dry ingredients with the liquid below. Next, stir in the milk and vanilla. When the batter is smooth (but not overmixed), stir in the sprinkles. Cook in the microwave for 2 to 2½ minutes, or until the cake looks done. It should not bubble over. Let the cake cool for a few minutes before eating.

1 egg

¼ cup (50 g) sugar

3 tablespoons (45 ml) canola oil

5 tablespoons (40 g) gluten-free low-FODMAP flour

⅛ teaspoon xanthan gum, if not added to your flour

⅛ teaspoon baking powder

Pinch of salt

3 tablespoons (45 ml) low-FODMAP milk (such as almond milk or lactose-free milk)

¼ teaspoon vanilla extract

1½ teaspoons candy sprinkles (rainbow or other colors)

NOTES

+ Using a whole egg for this recipe makes the cake too "eggy." One large egg is about 3¼ tablespoons (39 ml). Feel free to use a smaller egg so that you have less waste.

+ In a small cake like this, measurements really matter, so pay close attention to the ingredients (like xanthan gum) for the best texture.

VARIATION

+ Instead of sprinkles, try this with 1 tablespoon (9 g) semisweet chocolate chips!

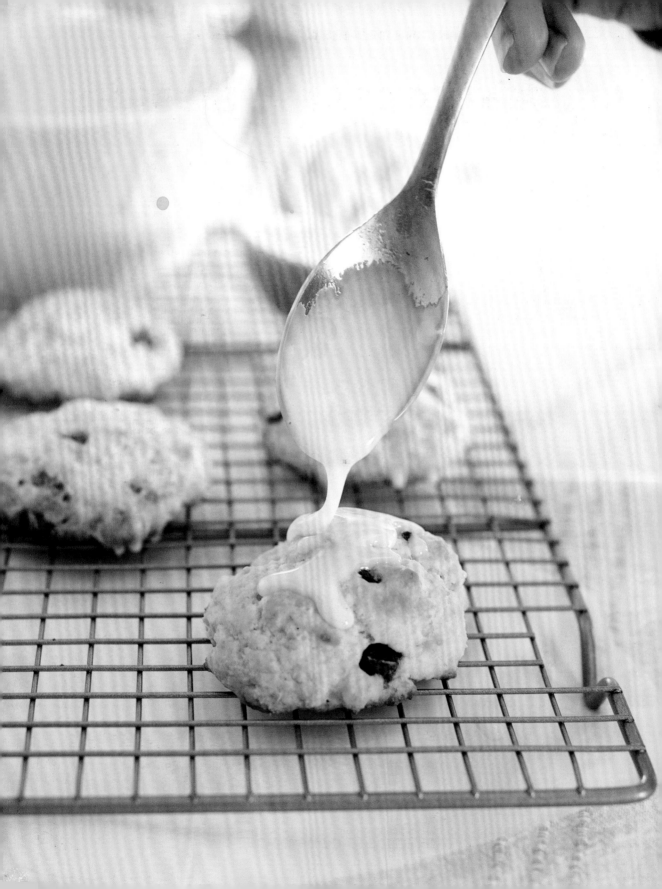

CHOCOLATE ORANGE BISCUITS WITH ORANGE GLAZE

These light and flaky biscuits can be served as a breakfast, snack, or dessert. The fresh orange provides delicious flavor and aroma, while the chocolate chips and sugary glaze make it a sweet treat. My friend told me these remind her of "cake batter cookies," but I think they taste more like scones. So good!

Preheat the oven to 400°F (200°C or gas mark 6) and place a rack in the center of the oven. Line a baking sheet with a baking mat or parchment paper or spray with nonstick cooking spray.

In a large mixing bowl, combine the pancake mix, sugar, and salt. Whisk the egg and milk in a separate glass or bowl. Add the vanilla and whisk again. Add the milk mixture to the dry mixture and stir. Add the melted butter and mix to incorporate (you may wish to use your hands). Knead in the chocolate chips and orange zest. Using a trigger ice cream scoop, portion out 15 biscuits onto the sheet. The dough may be crumbly; it is okay to smooth out the tops of the biscuits with your hands and flatten slightly. Bake for 12 to 14 minutes, or until golden. Remove the biscuits from the oven and let cool for 5 minutes.

In a small bowl, combine the orange juice and confectioners' sugar to create the orange glaze. Place the biscuits on a cooling rack and drizzle with the orange glaze. Serve immediately. These can also be chilled until ready to serve; reheat in a 250°F (120°C or gas mark ½) oven for 10 minutes.

Cooking spray (optional)

2 cups (240 g) all-purpose gluten-free pancake/biscuit mix (see Tip, page 44)

2 tablespoons (25 g) granulated sugar

½ teaspoon salt

1 egg

½ cup (120 ml) low-FODMAP milk (such as almond milk or lactose-free milk)

½ teaspoon vanilla extract

¼ cup (60 ml) melted unsalted butter

½ cup (75 g) semisweet chocolate chips

Zest and juice of 1 small orange (about 2 teaspoons [4 g] zest and 1 tablespoon [15 ml] juice)

1 cup (120 g) confectioners' sugar

VARIATION

+ Try this with blueberries or dried cranberries instead of chocolate chips for a different flavor.

INTENSELY ADDICTIVE CORNFLAKE COOKIES WITH CHOCOLATE CHIPS

These chewy cornflake cookies are absolutely delicious and incredibly addictive. When I bring them to work, they disappear in minutes. FODMAP fact: While high-fructose corn syrup is high-FODMAP, regular corn syrup is safe for the low-FODMAP diet.

½ cup (100 g) sugar

½ cup (120 ml) light corn syrup

½ cup (120 g) creamy salted almond butter (if using unsalted, add ¼ teaspoon salt)

½ teaspoon vanilla extract

2 cups (56 g) low-FODMAP cornflakes

½ cup (75 g) semisweet dairy-free chocolate chips

Line a baking sheet with parchment or wax paper and set aside.

In a large pot, combine the sugar, corn syrup, and almond butter. Cook over medium-low heat, stirring constantly, until just beginning to boil, making sure the sugar doesn't burn. As soon as the mixture begins to boil, remove from the heat and stir in the vanilla extract, salt (if using unsalted almond butter), and cornflakes. Stir by hand with a large spoon until the cornflakes are evenly coated in the almond butter mixture. Add the chocolate chips and stir (they will melt).

Use a small ice cream scoop to drop cookies onto the prepared baking sheet before the mixture starts to harden. Let cool at room temperature or in the refrigerator before eating. Store in a sealed container at room temperature.

NOTE Kellogg's Corn Flakes have been certified low-FODMAP, but are not gluten-free. Gluten-free brands of cornflakes with low-FODMAP ingredients include Nestlé Gluten Free Cornflakes and EnviroKidz Lightly Frosted Amazon Flakes. Be aware that many brands of gluten-free cornflakes contain fruit concentrates, and those should be avoided. You may find another brand in your area that is safe to enjoy.

VARIATION

+ If you are allergic to nuts, try sunflower seed butter in place of almond butter.

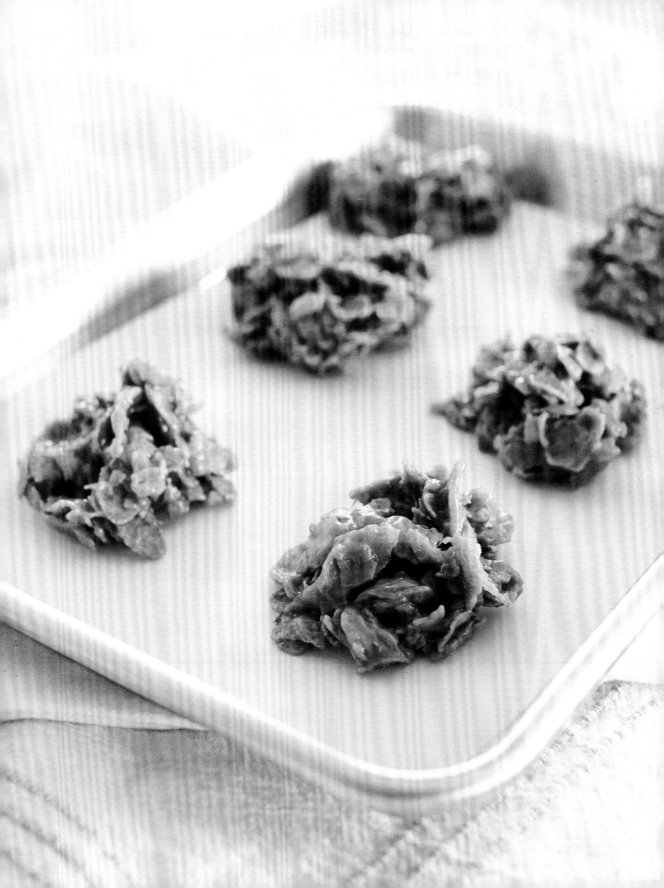

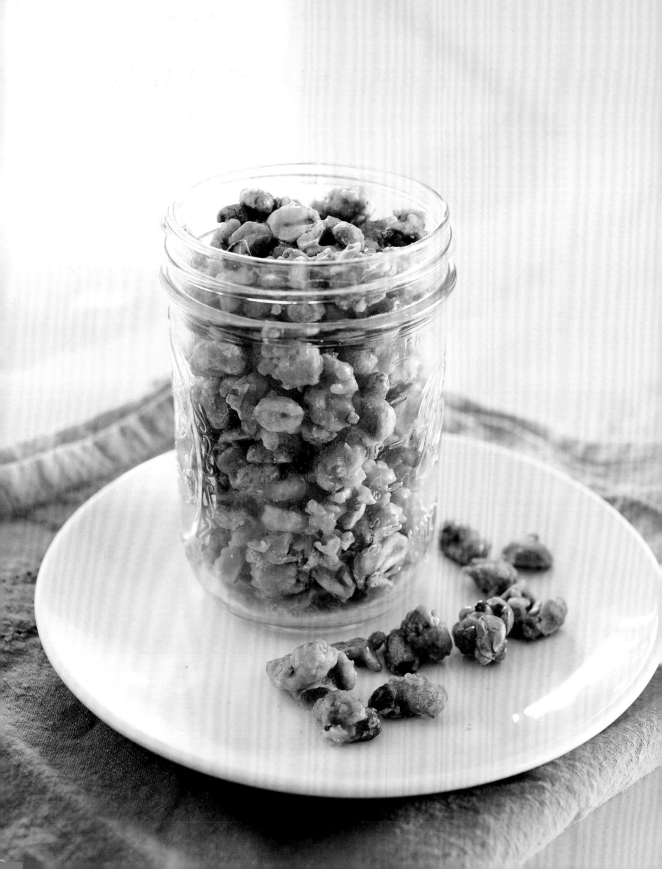

ONE-POT CANDIED PEANUTS

Candied peanuts are a wonderful snack choice, provided you eat a reasonable portion. Peanuts are full of healthy fats, fiber, and nutrition and are very inexpensive. Note that *dry-roasted* peanuts contain high-FODMAP additives like onion powder and other seasonings, and will not work for this recipe.

Line a baking sheet with wax or parchment paper. Place the peanuts, water, and sugar in a large pan or pot over low heat and cook until the sugar is melted. Stir constantly until the mixture thickens into a syrup, adjusting the heat as necessary so that the sugar doesn't burn; do not let it boil. The mixture will begin to change from clear to light amber in about 10 minutes. Be patient—it will happen. The liquid will suddenly become thicker and will be almost completely evaporated. At this point, stir until the peanuts are coated and appear glazed, then remove the pan from the heat. Sprinkle the salt over the nuts, if using.

Spread the peanuts on the prepared baking sheet into a single layer, gently separating with two forks, if necessary. When cooled completely, place the nuts in an airtight container, or separate into 1-ounce (28 g) servings and package individually.

NOTE These are very easy to make, but you will need to be patient. The key is to take it slow to avoid burning the sugar.

2 cups (250 g) unsalted roasted peanuts

⅓ cup (80 ml) water

1 cup (200 g) sugar

1 teaspoon flaky sea salt (optional)

MOUTHWATERING SNACKS AND TREATS

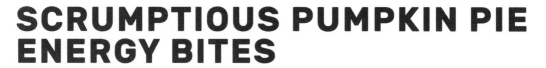

SCRUMPTIOUS PUMPKIN PIE ENERGY BITES

This is one of my favorite recipes for a versatile treat that is easy to whip up. Energy bites are the ideal snack to have mid-morning or after you hit the gym. The warm flavor of pumpkin is perfect any time of the year. But, if you aren't a fan of pumpkin, you can modify the recipe based on the variation below. FODMAP fact: Coconut is delicious, healthy, and low-FODMAP. You can enjoy ⅔ cup (64 g) of shredded coconut as one serving.

1 cup (80 g) traditional rolled oats

⅔ cup (64 g) unsweetened shredded coconut

½ cup (120 g) smooth salted almond butter (or add ½ teaspoon salt if using unsalted)

⅓ cup (85 g) canned pumpkin puree

½ cup (75 g) semisweet chocolate chips

¼ cup (60 ml) maple syrup

1 teaspoon vanilla extract

2 tablespoons (16 g) chia seeds

1 teaspoon pumpkin pie spice

Stir all the ingredients together in a medium bowl until thoroughly mixed. Cover and let chill in the refrigerator for 20 minutes, to make handling easier. Once chilled, roll into balls of about 1 inch (2.5 cm) diameter (a small cookie scoop works well). If needed, add more maple syrup or nut butter to achieve the desired consistency. Store in a sealed container in the refrigerator or freezer.

NOTE I eat these straight from the freezer, as the texture is still chewy and very refreshing.

VARIATION

+ If you don't like pumpkin, then remove the pumpkin puree and pumpkin spice and add 2 tablespoons (30 ml) more maple syrup and ¼ cup (32 g) ground flaxseeds.

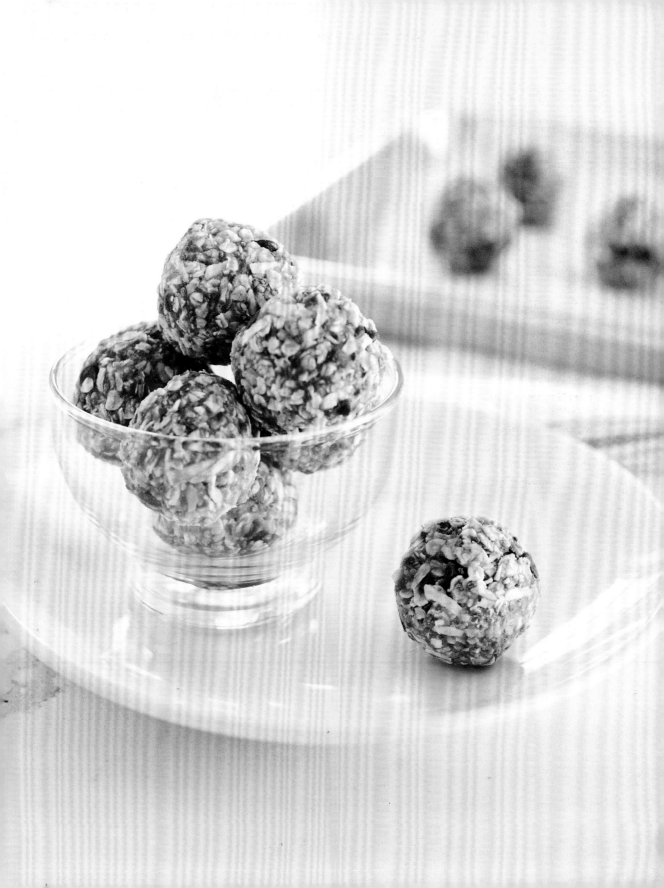

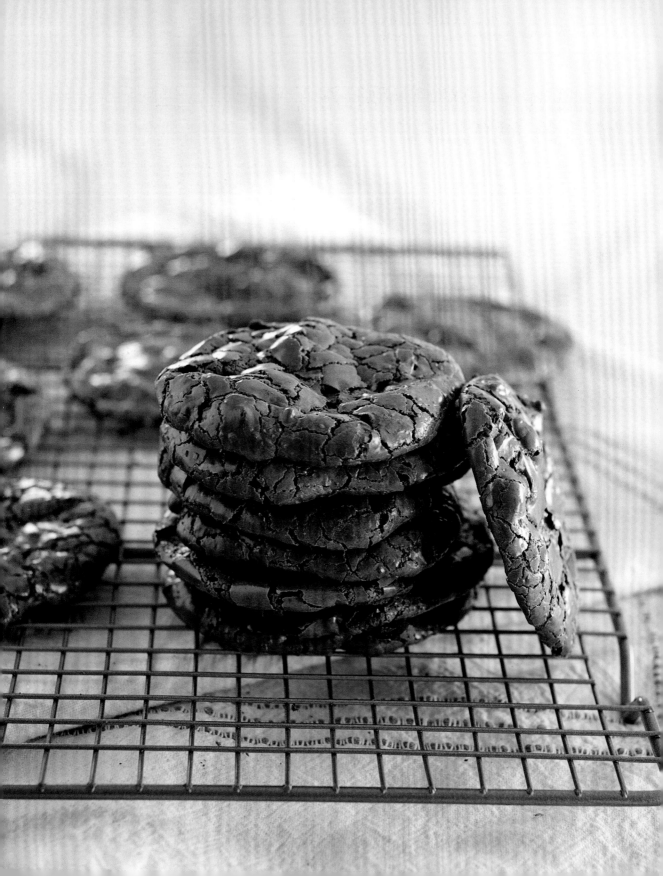

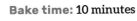
CHEWY BROWNIE COOKIES WITH WALNUTS

These chewy chocolate cookies are the BEST. You can mix them by hand, using one bowl, and they contain no flour or added fats. But they taste like a rich, fudge brownie. FODMAP fact: Walnuts are low-FODMAP in ¼-cup (30 g) servings.

Preheat the oven to 350°F (180°C or gas mark 4) and place a rack in the center of the oven. Line two baking sheets with parchment paper.

In a large bowl, combine the confectioners' sugar, cocoa powder, and salt. Add the egg whites and vanilla and blend by hand, forming a thick, sticky dough. If there is not enough egg white to make the dough scoopable, then add one more egg white. The dough should be thick, but not a dense paste. Stir in the walnuts. Drop the dough in small rounded spoonfuls onto the prepared sheets, leaving 2 inches (5 cm) between cookies. Bake for 10 minutes, or until they appear set; they will have a shiny surface with cracks. Let cool on the baking sheets. Store in the refrigerator or freezer.

2½ cups (300 g) confectioners' sugar

1 cup (120 g) unsweetened cocoa powder

⅛ teaspoon kosher salt

3 egg whites, or more as needed

2 teaspoons (10 ml) vanilla extract

1 cup (120 g) chopped toasted walnuts (page 40)

TIPS

+ To stick the parchment paper to the baking sheet, use a dab of the cookie batter underneath each corner.

+ To separate egg yolk from the white, crack the egg into half of its shell, or into your palm over a clear glass. Let the white collect into the glass beneath. Be careful not to get any yolk in the whites for best results.

VARIATION

+ Try 1 cup (150 g) of dairy-free chocolate chips instead of walnuts for an even more decadent treat.

CARROT MUG MUFFIN WITH WALNUTS AND COCONUT

This is a simple and delicious mug muffin that can be modified for a variety of stir-ins. Try it with the classic glaze recipe below. FODMAP fact: Carrots are a vegetable in which FODMAPs are not detected, so you can enjoy as many as you wish.

1 egg

¼ cup (50 g) sugar, plus more for sprinkling

3 tablespoons (45 ml) canola oil

3 tablespoons (25 g) finely grated or processed carrots (about 1 medium carrot)

5 tablespoons (40 g) gluten-free low-FODMAP flour

Pinch of salt

⅛ teaspoon xanthan gum (if not added to your flour choice)

⅛ teaspoon baking powder

½ teaspoon ground cinnamon, plus more for sprinkling

2 tablespoons (30 ml) low-FODMAP milk (such as almond milk or lactose-free milk)

½ teaspoon vanilla extract

1 tablespoon (9 g) toasted chopped walnuts (page 40)

1 tablespoon (5 g) shredded coconut (sweetened or unsweetened)

Crack the egg into a 16-ounce (450 ml) or larger microwave-safe mug, whisk, and remove 2 tablespoons (30 ml). Discard the remaining egg or set aside for another recipe. Add the sugar and whisk to combine. Add the oil, then the carrots, and stir to blend. In a small bowl, combine the flour, salt, xanthan gum, baking powder, and cinnamon. Add the flour mixture to the wet ingredients and stir to combine. Stir in the milk and vanilla. Fold in the walnuts and coconut and sprinkle with additional cinnamon and sugar, if desired. Microwave on high for 2 minutes 30 seconds to 2 minutes 45 seconds, watching so that it doesn't bubble over. Serve immediately.

TIP *Bonus recipe!* For a simple low-FODMAP vanilla glaze, combine ½ cup (60 g) confectioners' sugar with 1 to 3 teaspoons (5 to 15 ml) low-FODMAP milk and ¼ teaspoon vanilla extract; drizzle over the cake if desired.

VARIATION

+ If you like more spice, add ¼ teaspoon ground nutmeg and a pinch of ground ginger, or use 1 to 2 teaspoons pumpkin pie spice instead.

MAPLE AND CINNAMON PROTEIN YOGURT

This is one of my favorite midafternoon treats; it keeps me from reaching for sugary snacks. Protein yogurt is absolutely delicious, full of nutrients, and very inexpensive. Add 1 tablespoon (15 g) of almond butter for even more protein and healthy fats.

Combine all the ingredients in a bowl and enjoy immediately.

NOTE Top with fruit, toasted coconut, or chocolate chips, if desired.

1 cup (120 g) plain low-FODMAP yogurt (such as coconut yogurt or lactose-free yogurt)

2 tablespoons (30 ml) maple syrup

½ teaspoon ground cinnamon

1 tablespoon (8 g) low-FODMAP protein powder

   Yield: 4 servings   **Prep time: 10 minutes**   **Passive chill time: 3 hours or overnight**

CHOCOLATE AND CINNAMON CHIA SEED PUDDING

This chia seed pudding is so much better than regular pudding. The chia seeds give great texture, not to mention fiber, protein and healthy fats. Plus, each tablespoon (8 g) of cocoa powder contains an additional 2 grams of fiber and 1 gram of protein. A super-healthy and delicious dessert!

Place the milk, maple syrup, cocoa powder, and cinnamon in a large glass and use an immersion blender to combine well. Add the chia seeds and blend again. Let stand for about 5 minutes and stir again to ensure the chia seeds don't settle to the bottom of the glass. Cover and place in the refrigerator for 3 hours or overnight, until the chia seeds swell.

2 cups (480 ml) low-FODMAP milk (such as almond milk or lactose-free milk)

3 tablespoons (45 ml) maple syrup

3 tablespoons (24 g) cocoa powder

½ teaspoon ground cinnamon

½ cup (60 g) chia seeds

VARIATION

+ Try this with ½ teaspoon espresso powder instead of cinnamon for a mocha flavor.

CRUNCHY KALE CHIPS WITH LEMON

So much better than potato chips, these kale chips are crispy, crunchy, and delicious. I love making this snack as a healthy option for the kids after school or when watching the game on TV. FODMAP fact: Trace levels of FODMAPs are noted in kale, so you can eat as much as you wish.

1 bunch curly kale, stemmed and torn or chopped into roughly 2-inch (5 cm) square pieces (about 6 cups [370 g])

3 tablespoons (45 ml) olive oil

1 tablespoon (18 g) flaky sea salt, plus more to taste

1 lemon, cut into wedges

Preheat the oven to 350°F (180°C or gas mark 4) and place a rack in the center of the oven. Line two baking sheets with parchment paper or silicone baking mats.

Spread the kale on the baking sheets and ensure leaves are completely dry. Rub each leaf lightly with the olive oil. Sprinkle with the salt. Bake until crispy but still green, 12 to 15 minutes. Remove from the oven and squeeze over the fresh lemon juice. Add more salt to taste.

NOTE These are crispiest the day they are made, but they can also be stored at room temperature in a covered container.

VARIATION

+ If you like a kick to your chips, then sprinkle with red pepper flakes after baking.

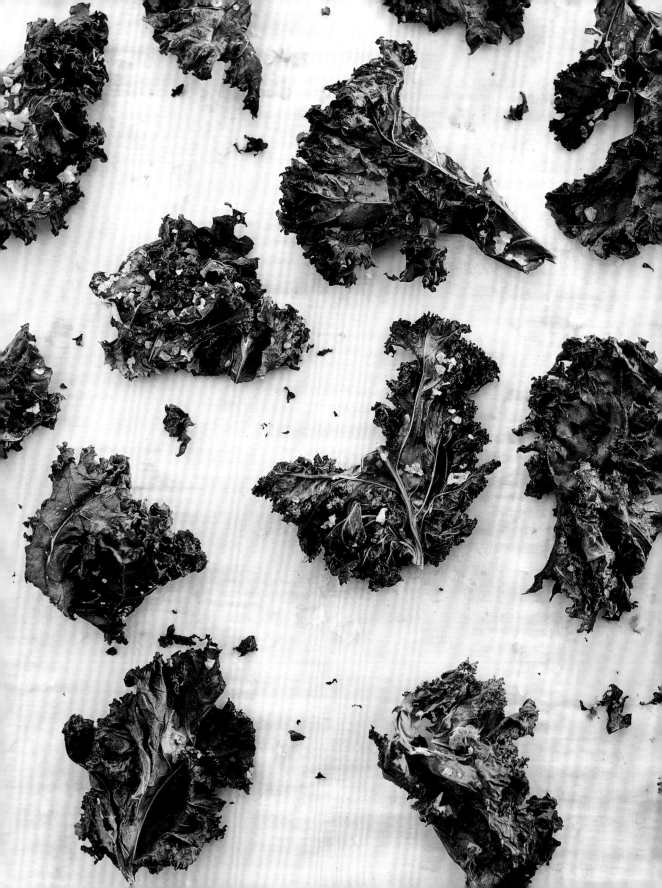

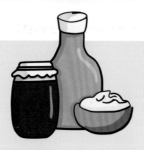

8

AMAZING STOCKS, SAUCES, DRESSINGS, AND DIPS

Your food will have plenty of flavor with these recipes for low-FODMAP stocks, sauces, dressings, and dips. Easy and delicious!

SENSATIONAL SOY MAPLE DRESSING

This dressing combines perfectly with my Kale and Cabbage Salad with Pepitas (page 58) and my Warm Quinoa and Spinach Salad (page 61). But don't stop there! Try it as a marinade for fish or chicken, or drizzle it over steamed rice.

Combine all the ingredients in a large jar and shake to blend well. Store in the refrigerator for 2 to 3 days.

VARIATION

+ If you don't have maple syrup, you can use light corn syrup or granulated sugar.

¼ cup (60 ml) olive oil

¼ cup (60 ml) rice vinegar (not seasoned rice vinegar, as that has sugar added)

3 tablespoons (45 ml) tamari (gluten-free soy sauce) or soy sauce

2 tablespoons (30 ml) maple syrup

Salt and pepper to taste

   Yield: 3 cups (720 g), or 16 to 24 servings (2 to 3 tablespoons [30 to 45 g] each)
Prep time: 10 minutes

"HUMM IN YOUR HEAD" HUMMUS

This hummus will make your feet tap and your mouth smile. While chickpeas and garlic in typical recipes make hummus a big no-no for the low-FODMAP diet, this version uses canned chickpeas and infused oil. It is super easy and tastes sensational. Try it in my Hummus Pizza with Greek Salad (page 129). FODMAP fact: Tahini is low-FODMAP in 1-tablespoon (20 g) servings.

Place all the ingredients in a food processor and process to a smooth puree, adding water, 1 teaspoon at a time, if needed to adjust the consistency. Taste and adjust the seasoning as needed. Serve, garnished with extra paprika and infused oil. Store in a resealable container in the refrigerator for up to 1 week.

NOTE Tahini is a paste made from sesame seeds. Select a tahini that contains only ground sesame seeds and their oil to ensure it is low-FODMAP.

One 15-ounce (420 g) can chickpeas, drained

½ cup (120 g) tahini (sesame paste), with some of its oil

¼ cup (60 ml) garlic-infused olive oil (page 25), plus extra for drizzling

1 tablespoon (7 g) paprika, plus extra for garnish

2 tablespoons (30 ml) freshly squeezed lemon juice (about ½ medium lemon)

Salt and pepper to taste

159

RED WINE MARINARA

I am obsessed with this marinara sauce. It is rich and robust due to the red wine, and you can personalize the sweetness to your taste. Zucchini is a wonderful addition to this marinara sauce, because it adds texture, color, and delicious flavor. FODMAP fact: You can enjoy ⅓ cup (65 g) sliced zucchini per low-FODMAP serving.

2 tablespoons (30 ml) garlic-infused olive oil (page 25)

½ cup (60 g) finely chopped carrot

½ cup (75 g) diced zucchini

One 15-ounce (420 g) can diced tomatoes

One 15-ounce (420 g) can tomato sauce or pureed tomatoes (see Tip)

6 tablespoons (90 g) tomato paste

¾ cup (180 ml) dry red wine

2 teaspoons low-FODMAP Italian seasoning, homemade (page 49) or store-bought

¼ cup (50 g) sugar, or to taste (optional)

Salt and pepper to taste

Heat the infused oil in a large saucepan over medium-low heat, add the carrot, and cook until translucent but not browned, about 5 minutes. Stir in the zucchini and cook until the veggies are cooked through, about 5 minutes. Pour in the diced tomatoes and bring the mixture to a boil, stirring often. Pour in the tomato sauce and bring to a simmer. Let the sauce simmer until slightly thickened and bubbling, stirring occasionally, about 10 minutes. Stir in the tomato paste and wine. Bring the sauce back to a simmer, and stir in the Italian seasoning, sugar (if using), salt, and pepper. Simmer until the seasonings are blended and the sauce is heated through, about 3 more minutes. May be refrigerated in jar(s) for up to 1 month.

NOTE A small quantity of wine will enhance the flavor of your sauce. During cooking, the alcohol in the wine evaporates, but the sweetness and acid notes remain.

TIP If you can't find tomato sauce without onion or garlic, then you can make sauce from canned tomato paste using a 1:1 ratio with water. It works like a charm!

RESTAURANT-STYLE SALSA

Salsa is a low-calorie condiment that is a staple in our home. Making it from scratch gives it a fresh flavor just like the one at your favorite restaurant, but without the onion or garlic. This salsa is so delicious with Beef and Spinach Enchiladas (page 100), Cheese and Spinach Quesadillas (page 123), and corn chips. It tastes even better made a day ahead.

Heat the oil in a pan or small pot over medium heat. Add the canned tomatoes, chile, cilantro, salt, and lime juice and stir to combine. Bring to a boil and then decrease the heat to low. Add the sugar to taste, if desired. Simmer for 15 minutes. Allow to cool, then store in the refrigerator in a covered jar for up to 10 days.

NOTE For mild salsa, use ½ chile; for medium salsa, use 1 chile.

TIP If you don't have fresh cilantro, substitute 1 tablespoon (1 g) dried cilantro.

2 tablespoons (30 ml) garlic-infused olive oil (page 25)

One 15-ounce (420 g) can diced tomatoes, no seasonings added

½ to 1 red chile pepper (see Note), seeded and chopped

8 sprigs fresh cilantro

½ teaspoon salt

2 tablespoons (30 ml) freshly squeezed lime juice (about 1 lime)

1 to 2 teaspoons sugar (optional)

VARIATION

+ Add 1 teaspoon ground cumin or use a serrano chile instead of the red chile for a different flavor and color.

HERBY TOFU VEGAN RICOTTA

This tofu "ricotta" reminds me of herbed cream cheese. I love it spread on rice cakes with pumpkin seeds and olive oil drizzled on top. Try it in my Herby Ricotta and Vegetable Hoagie (page 126)!

One 14-ounce (392 g) package extra-firm tofu, drained

2 tablespoons (2 g) nutritional yeast, plus more as desired

¼ cup (60 ml) freshly squeezed lemon juice (about 1 lemon)

1 tablespoon (15 ml) garlic-infused olive oil (page 25)

¾ cup (28 g) roughly chopped fresh basil

Salt and pepper to taste

1 teaspoon sugar (optional)

Add the tofu, nutritional yeast, lemon juice, and oil to a blender or food processor and process until smooth. Add the basil and pulse a few times to combine. Season with salt and pepper to taste and add sugar or additional yeast, if desired. Can be stored in the refrigerator for up to 1 week.

NOTE For a stronger cheese flavor, add more nutritional yeast to taste.

ASIAN PEANUT DRESSING

This rich, peanutty dressing is wonderful over Peanut Pad Thai (page 130), salads, or crispy tofu (page 133). FODMAP fact: Hot sauces are safe on the low-FODMAP diet, but many people with IBS find spicy foods to be a trigger. Feel free to omit it, if you are sensitive.

¼ cup (60 ml) canola oil

1 tablespoon (15 ml) tamari (gluten-free soy sauce) or soy sauce

3 tablespoons (45 g) brown sugar

3 tablespoons (45 g) smooth natural peanut butter

1 tablespoon (15 ml) freshly squeezed lime juice (about ½ lime)

1 tablespoon (15 ml) rice vinegar

1 tablespoon (15 ml) light corn syrup

1 teaspoon hot sauce

1 teaspoon grated fresh ginger

Combine all the ingredients in a mason jar or other container and whisk well to blend. Store in the refrigerator for up to 1 week.

VARIATION

+ If you don't have fresh ginger, substitute ½ teaspoon ground ginger.

Yield: 2 cups (480 ml), or 10 to 16 servings (2 to 3 tablespoons [30 to 45 ml] each)
Prep time: 5 minutes   **Cook time:** 15 to 20 minutes

BOLD BBQ SAUCE

This BBQ sauce recipe is adjustable to your preference for sweet or spicy, and cooks up in a snap. FODMAP fact: Many chili powders contain onion or garlic additives. Read labels, and make sure you select pure ancho chile powder for this recipe.

Combine all the ingredients in a medium saucepan and stir well. Cook over medium-high heat for 15 to 20 minutes, until thickened. Adjust the spices to taste. Allow to cool and then transfer to a jar or resealable container. Refrigerate until ready to use, or for up to 1 week. This tastes better made a day ahead.

NOTE This recipe is wonderful with my BBQ Tofu "Steaks" (page 122).

1 cup (240 g) tomato paste

½ cup (120 ml) corn syrup

½ cup (120 ml) water

1 tablespoon (7 g) ancho chile powder, or to taste

¼ cup (60 ml) distilled white vinegar

¼ cup (60 ml) tamari (gluten-free soy sauce) or soy sauce

2 tablespoons (30 g) brown sugar

Yield: 3 cups (730 ml), or 24 servings (2 tablespoons [30 ml] each)
Prep time: 2 minutes   **Cook time:** 10 minutes

MICROWAVE SWEET AND SOUR SAUCE

This is a tangy sauce that is perfect on chicken nuggets (page 104), tofu nuggets (page 133), vegetables, or rice. FODMAP fact: One 0.3-ounce packet (13 g) of ketchup is one low-FODMAP serving.

Combine the ketchup, vinegar, water, and sugars in a large microwave-safe bowl. Stir well. Microwave uncovered on high for 3 minutes, then stop to stir again. Microwave for another 3 to 4 minutes, or until boiling. Remove from the microwave and stir the cornstarch/water mixture into the sauce. Microwave for another 3 minutes, until thickened. Let cool, then transfer to a jar or resealable container and store in the refrigerator for up to 1 week.

NOTE You can also make this on the stovetop over medium-low heat.

½ cup (120 g) ketchup (no high-fructose corn syrup)

½ cup (120 ml) distilled white vinegar

¾ cup (180 ml) water

1¼ cups (250 g) granulated sugar

½ cup (120 g) lightly packed brown sugar

3 tablespoons (24 g) cornstarch, dissolved in ¼ cup (60 ml) cold water

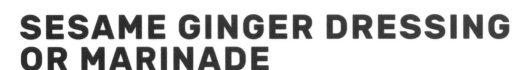

SESAME GINGER DRESSING OR MARINADE

Have you ever tried an Asian salad made with thin sliced carrots and chopped lettuce, topped with a yummy ginger dressing? Here is the recipe for the dressing . . . it's so delicious, I want to lick the bowl. It is also a wonderful marinade for chicken or fish. Try it with my Sesame Ginger Tempeh Stir-Fry (page 132).

2 tablespoons (16 g) grated fresh ginger

2 tablespoons (30 ml) sesame oil

3 tablespoons (45 ml) rice vinegar (not seasoned rice vinegar, as that has sugar added)

¼ cup (60 ml) tamari (gluten-free soy sauce) or soy sauce

3 tablespoons (45 ml) maple syrup

1 tablespoon (15 g) tahini

1 tablespoon (15 ml) garlic-infused olive oil (page 25)

2 tablespoons (30 ml) olive oil

Combine all the ingredients in a bowl or jar and whisk or shake until smooth. Store in the refrigerator for up to 1 week.

NOTE If this doesn't combine well by hand, then try using an immersion blender.

VARIATION

+ Skip the tahini altogether, or try with your favorite nut butter instead.

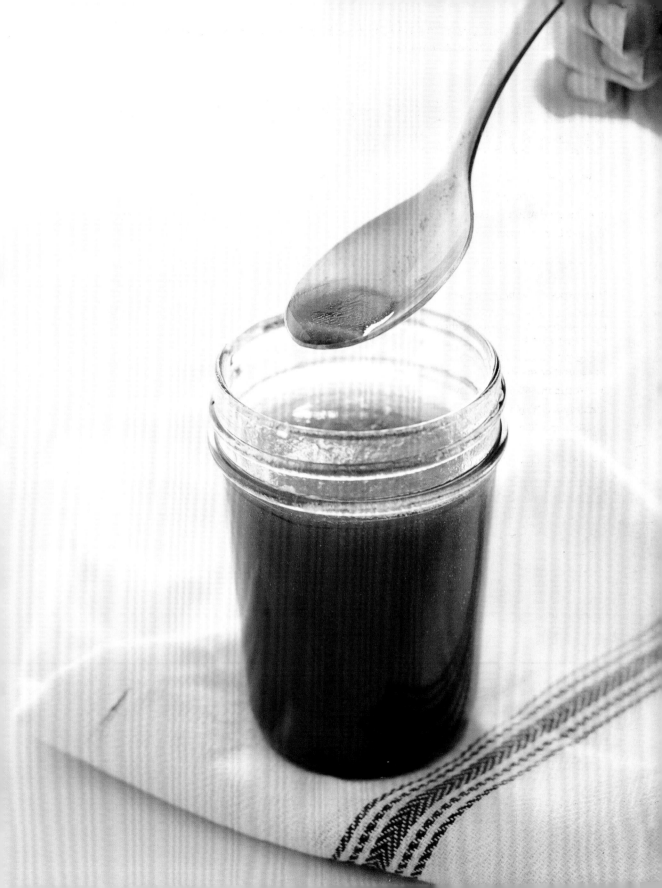

KALE AND BASIL PESTO WITH WALNUTS

I love a good pesto, and this recipe is one of my favorites. Kale provides a deep flavor, which is perfectly balanced by the toasted walnuts, fresh herbs, and infused oil. It goes wonderfully drizzled over low-FODMAP focaccia, pasta, or crackers. Try it in my Pesto Penne with Tofu (page 127). I like to massage the kale leaves after chopping, because it softens the kale and improves the flavor.

4 cups (268 g) chopped kale, stemmed

¼ cup (30 g) chopped toasted walnuts (page 40)

1 cup (40 g) fresh basil leaves

1 tablespoon (1 g) nutritional yeast

1 tablespoon (15 ml) freshly squeezed lemon juice (about ½ small lemon)

¾ teaspoon salt, plus more to taste

Freshly ground pepper to taste

5 tablespoons (75 ml) olive oil

1 tablespoon (15 ml) garlic-infused olive oil (page 25)

Place the kale in a blender or food processor and process for 20 to 30 seconds, until broken down. Add the walnuts, basil, nutritional yeast, lemon juice, salt, and pepper and pulse to combine. Slowly drizzle in the oils, one at a time, while the food processor is running. Blend for 30 seconds to 1 minute, until the kale is well blended and the pesto is thickened, scraping down the sides if necessary. Taste, and add more salt and pepper if desired. Store in the refrigerator for up to 5 days.

VARIATIONS

+ Try this with spinach instead of kale.

+ Add some fresh rosemary or oregano!

HOMEMADE CHICKEN STOCK USING A SLOW COOKER

Homemade chicken stock is packed with nutrients, protein, and natural collagen. It is wonderful for boosting immunity, promoting gut health, and providing building blocks for your skin and hair. There's a reason we use it as a remedy when we are sick!

Place the chicken pieces in a 5- or 6-quart (4.5 to 5.4 L) slow cooker. Add enough water to cover with about ½ inch (1.3 cm) left at the top (this may be 8 cups [1.8 L] or more). Add the seasonings and chopped carrot. Cook on low for 12 to 15 hours (overnight is good). Strain the stock and discard the chicken pieces, herbs, and carrot. The stock may be used immediately or frozen in individual serving sizes after cooling.

NOTE I make this stock once per month and store it in 1-cup (240 ml) servings in the freezer, so it is always ready for cooking.

3 pounds (1365 g) chicken wings or thighs

1 tablespoon (5 g) black peppercorns (not ground pepper)

1 tablespoon (18 g) salt

1 bay leaf

1 teaspoon dried thyme

1 teaspoon dried parsley or 1 bunch fresh parsley

1 medium carrot, peeled and chopped

VARIATION
+ Add some other herbs, such as rosemary, sage, or dill.

CREAMY POPPYSEED SALAD DRESSING

This creamy dressing is sweet and tangy. I love it so much that I use it to dip fruit as well. Enjoy this with my Summertime Salad with Toasted Pecans (page 62). FODMAP fact: Poppyseeds are a great source of fiber and are low-FODMAP in servings of 2 tablespoons (24 g).

¼ cup (60 ml) red wine vinegar

5 tablespoons (60 g) sugar

1 tablespoon poppyseeds

½ teaspoon salt

½ teaspoon ground mustard powder

½ cup (120 ml) olive oil

2 teaspoons (10 g) full-fat mayonnaise or vegan mayonnaise (page 68)

In a bowl, whisk the red wine vinegar and sugar until the sugar is mostly dissolved. Add the poppyseeds, salt, and ground mustard and whisk to combine. Whisking steadily, pour the oil into the dressing in a slow stream. Continue whisking until completely combined. Add the mayonnaise and whisk again. Transfer to a covered container and store in the refrigerator for up to 1 week.

TIP An immersion blender works well instead of whisking by hand.

THE BEST RANCH DRESSING OR DIP

Ranch is the most popular dip in the United States, and this recipe is the best I have tried. I use it for French fries, vegetables, and (my favorite) potato chips. Dipping chips in this ranch reminds me of "sour cream and onion" flavor. FODMAP fact: The green tip of the scallion is low-FODMAP, provided you avoid the rest of the stalk.

1 teaspoon garlic-infused olive oil (page 25), or more as needed

¼ cup (15 g) finely chopped fresh parsley

2 tablespoons (8 g) chopped chives or green scallion tips

1 cup (240 g) full-fat mayonnaise or vegan mayonnaise (page 68)

½ cup (120 g) low-FODMAP yogurt (such as coconut yogurt or lactose-free yogurt) or lactose-free sour cream

Salt and pepper to taste

Combine all the ingredients in a mason jar or bottle and shake well. Store in the refrigerator for up to 5 days.

TIP If you don't have fresh parsley, you can use 1 tablespoon (1.3 g) dried parsley, but the texture and flavor will be slightly different.

COPYCAT SECRET SAUCE

I have never had the pleasure of enjoying Shake Shack sauce, but my family raves about it. Making it at home means I can ensure it isn't high in FODMAPs. Their recipe calls for pickle brine, but many pickles contain onion and garlic. So, I substituted the brine from capers. If you can access pickles without onion and garlic, then feel free to use that instead. FODMAP fact: Capers are low-FODMAP in 1-tablespoon (8 g) servings.

Combine all the ingredients in a bowl or bottle and mix well. Store in the refrigerator for up to 5 days.

NOTE Capers are the seed of a plant commonly grown in Europe and are used in many Mediterranean recipes.

TIP Try this sauce over The Best Burgers (page 108) or with Crispy Chicken Nuggets (page 104).

½ cup (120 g) full-fat mayonnaise or vegan mayonnaise (page 68)

1 tablespoon (11 g) Dijon mustard

¾ teaspoon ketchup

¼ teaspoon brine from jar of capers

Pinch of cayenne pepper

EVERYONE'S FAVORITE ITALIAN DRESSING

Italian dressing is a classic for tossed salads, baked potatoes, or grilled vegetables. This recipe tastes *so* much better than store-bought and is made with ingredients you have in your pantry already. Check out my bonus recipe below for easy Italian chicken dinner!

Combine all the ingredients in a large bottle and shake vigorously to emulsify. Store in the refrigerator for up to 1 week. Tastes best made a day ahead.

TIP *Bonus recipe!* For Italian chicken breasts, place raw chicken breasts in a freezer bag and add the dressing (1 ounce [30 ml] of dressing for every 4 ounces [112 g] of chicken). Refrigerate for 30 minutes or up to overnight. Then grill on the barbecue (or broil in the oven) for 5 to 8 minutes per side, until cooked through.

½ cup (120 ml) red wine vinegar

¾ cup (180 ml) olive oil

¼ cup (60 ml) garlic-infused olive oil (page 25)

4 teaspoons (16 g) sugar, or to taste

2 teaspoons low-FODMAP Italian seasoning, homemade (page 49) or store-bought

¼ teaspoon red pepper flakes

Salt and pepper to taste

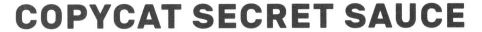

AMAZING STOCKS, SAUCES, DRESSINGS, AND DIPS

REFERENCES

References are listed in order of appearance in text.

CHAPTER 1

Saha, L. (2014). Irritable bowel syndrome: pathogenesis, diagnosis, treatment, and evidence-based medicine. *World Journal of Gastroenterology* 20, 6759–73.

Pauls, R. N., and Max, J. B. (2019). Symptoms and dietary practices of irritable bowel syndrome patients compared to controls: Results of a USA national survey. *Minerva Gastroenteroogica Dietologica* 65, 1–10.

Eswaran, S., Chey, W. D., Jackson, K., Pillai, S., Chey, S. W., and Han-Markey, T. (2017). A diet low in fermentable oligo-, di-, and monosaccharides and polyols improves quality of life and reduces activity impairment in patients with irritable bowel syndrome and diarrhea. *Clinical Gastroenterology and Hepatology* 15, 1890–99.

Major, G., Pritchard, S., Murray, K., Paul Alappadan, J., Hoad, C., Marciani, L., Gowland, P., and Spiller, R. (2016). Colon hypersensitivity to distension, rather than excessive gas production, produces carbohydrate-related symptoms in individuals with irritable bowel syndrome. *Gastroenterology* 152, 124–33.

Gibson, P. R., and Shepherd, S. J. (2012). Food choice as a key management strategy for functional gastrointestinal symptoms. *American Journal of Gastroenterology* 107, 657–66, quiz 667.

Hayes, P., Corish, C., O'Mahony, E., and Quigley, E. M. (2014). A dietary survey of patients with irritable bowel syndrome. *Journal of Human Nutrition and Dietetics* 27, Suppl 2, 36–47.

Varju, P., Farkas, N., Hegyi, P., Garami, A., Szabo, I., Illes, A., Solymar, M., Vincze, A., Balasko, M., Par, G., Bajor, J., Szucs, A., Huszar, O., Pecsi, D., and Czimmer, J. (2017). Low fermentable oligosaccharides, disaccharides, monosaccharides and polyols (FODMAP) diet improves symptoms in adults suffering from irritable bowel syndrome (IBS) compared to standard IBS diet: A meta-analysis of clinical studies. *PLoS One* 12, e0182942.

Pellissier, S., and Bonaz, B. (2017). The place of stress and emotions in the irritable bowel syndrome. *Vitamins and Hormones* 103, 327–54.

Marchesi, J. R., Adams, D. H., Fava, F., Hermes, G. D., Hirschfield, G. M., Hold, G., Quraishi, M. N., Kinross, J., Smidt, H., Tuohy, K. M., Thomas, L. V., Zoetendal, E. G., and Hart, A. (2016). The gut microbiota and host health: A new clinical frontier. *Gut* 65, 330–39.

Eswaran, S., Farida, J. P., Green, J., Miller, J. D., and Chey, W. D. (2017). Nutrition in the management of gastrointestinal diseases and disorders: The evidence for the low FODMAP diet. *Current Opinion in Pharmacology* 37, 151–57.

CHAPTER 3

Whelan, K., Martin, L. D., Staudacher, H. M., and Lomer, M. C. E. (2018). The low FODMAP diet in the management of irritable bowel syndrome: An evidence-based review of FODMAP restriction, reintroduction and personalisation in clinical practice. *Journal of Human Nutrition and Dietetics* 31, 239–55.

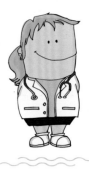

RESOURCES

FODMAP EVERYDAY
Information and low-FODMAP recipes.
www.fodmapeveryday.com

INTERNATIONAL FOUNDATION FOR GASTROINTESTINAL DISORDERS
A reliable and comprehensive source of support and information.
www.aboutibs.org

KATE SCARLATA
Kate Scarlata is a medical dietitian and expert in the low-FODMAP diet.
www.katescarlata.com

MONASH UNIVERSITY
Source for large volume of low-FODMAP research and creators of the Monash University Low-FODMAP Application.
www.monashfodmap.com

PATSY CATSOS
Patsy Catsos is a medical dietitian and expert in the low-FODMAP diet.
www.ibsfree.net

RACHEL PAULS FOOD
My website containing useful medical information as well as over 350 free low-FODMAP recipes.
www.rachelpaulsfood.com

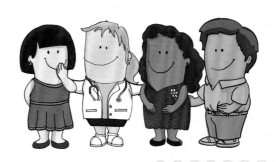

ACKNOWLEDGMENTS

THIS BOOK WOULD NOT HAVE BEEN POSSIBLE WITHOUT THE FOLLOWING PEOPLE:

Suzette Olson: The best low-FODMAP recipe tester in the world, and an important colleague for over a decade.

My husband, Cory: In work and in life, you are the person who cheers me on, has my back, and takes every curve in the road right next to me. I'm so lucky to have you.

My children, Hannah, Jack, and Zev: Three incredible people. I love you with everything I am. You show me the true meaning of joy and inspire me every day.

My mother, Jeanne: The person who shares my passion for reading and writing, and who never got bored hearing about this project.

The Rachel Pauls Food Team, with special thanks to John Rice: A fantastic group of talented individuals. Together we have built something that is enabling people to live healthier and happier lives.

My work family: Amazing partners, nurses, support staff, and fellows (past and present). You motivate me to strive to the highest standards.

Amanda Waddell and Quarto Publishing Group: The best partners I could have imagined in the making of this book.

ABOUT THE AUTHOR

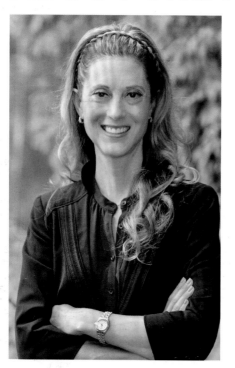

Dr. Rachel Pauls is an internationally renowned surgeon and medical researcher who is also a passionate chef and FODMAP blogger. She has published more than 100 original medical journal articles and book chapters, and currently serves as the program director for the Fellowship Program in Female Pelvic Medicine and Reconstructive Surgery. She is also director of research for the Division of Urogynecology at TriHealth, in Cincinnati.

An IBS sufferer, Dr. Pauls follows the low-FODMAP diet to successfully eliminate her own IBS symptoms. In order to help other people improve their IBS and other digestive issues, Dr. Pauls founded Rachel Pauls Food (www.rachelpaulsfood.com), one of the world's leading makers of delicious certified low-FODMAP food.

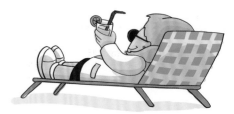

INDEX